Holistic Mental Health
Revised

A COMPARISON OF TRADITIONAL TREATMENTS AND
ALTERNATIVE TREATMENTS FOR MENTAL DISORDERS

DR. DAVE DISANO

iUniverse, Inc.
New York   Bloomington

Holistic Mental Health- Revised
A Comparison of Traditional Treatments and
Alternative Treatments for Mental Disorders

iUniverse books may be ordered through booksellers or by contacting:

iUniverse
1663 Liberty Drive
Bloomington, IN 47403
www.iuniverse.com
1-800-Authors (1-800-288-4677)

ISBN: 978-1-4401-5196-5 (pbk)
ISBN: 978-1-4401-5197-2 (ebk)

Printed in the United States of America

iUniverse rev. date: 7/14/2009

Disclaimer

This book contains *suggestions* on treatment for mental disorders, that the reader should be aware that, are in fact, suggestions only. Treatment for medical conditions should always be conducted by your healthcare professional. According to the FDA only physicians are allowed to prescribe medications, and the suggestions in this book are for dietary changes and/or supplements only. I am not a physician, and I am not prescribing any treatments in this book. *Holistic Mental Health-Revised* is reporting research by the medical and alternative health fields.

The reader should also be aware that supplements such as vitamins, minerals and herbs can interact with medications. They could have contradictory reactions (negative) or complimentary reactions (increase) with prescription medications. The reader should always consult with someone knowledgeable of such interactions before changing what you are taking.

DEDICATION

To my sunshine, my divine angel,
my soul matey, my eternal traveler;

Mary

Preface

Holistic Mental Health was initially intended as an unbiased look at treatments in mental health. I conducted the majority of the research for this book when writing my dissertation to complete my Ph.D. My dissertation was entitled *A Comparison of Allopathic and Naturopathic Treatments for Mental Disorders.* In it, I attempted to compare traditional western treatment (allopathic medicine) with alternative, and eastern (naturopathic medicine) for mental disorders such as Alzheimer's disease, anxiety, AD/HD, depression, headaches and migraines. However, the outcome of the research resulted in *Holistic Mental Health*, that in fact, is biased toward alternative treatment for mental disorders.

This bias is largely due to the overwhelming evidence of the negative effects of traditional western medicine, and the lack of a cure for the illness western medicine provides. Whereas, the naturopathic approach rarely has negative side effects in treatment, and focuses on curing the aliment. This is the difference between traditional Western medicine and Eastern medicine. Western medicine attempts to cure a disorder by treating the symptoms. Contrary to Eastern medicine that endeavors to cure by healing the body and finding the cause of the disorder. In most cases when you are treating the body with drugs, the drugs cause side effects that in some cases, may be far worse than the disease symptoms. The recent realization that many arthritis medications cause heart attacks is an example of drug side effects that are worse than the disease itself. Or, a popular medication used for ADHD was pulled off the market (February, 2005) in Canada due to connections with it causing seizures and heart attacks. Interestingly, in the U.S., the FDA only issued a warning!

My interest in holistic health started when I was in high school. At that time I noticed that the large abrasions on my arms that occurred from being a lineman on my high school football team would heal in half the normal time when I was taking large doses of vitamin C. I also noticed far fewer colds during wrestling season when I was hardly eating. Years later as a biochemistry teacher I came to appreciate how relatively young the science of biochemistry is. All the major discoveries of vitamins and the function of minerals in the body has occurred in the past hundred years. Vitamin A was first identified in 1913, named in 1920 (A for being the first discovered), and chemically isolated in 1931, by Swiss researcher Paul Karrar, who received a Nobel prize for his effort. New findings on the role and function of vitamins and minerals are continually in the news today.

The use of herbs to heal and cure the body date back thousands of years. Today consumers are demanding more information on these ancient miracle cures and Western medicine is appearing to make an attempt to satisfy that demand, if only in an effort to discredit herbal medicine's effectiveness. However, consumers are finding that the alternative approach can be just as effective, without the harmful, or even deadly side-effects of prescription medications. More and more people are taking the imitative for their own health, rather than blindly trust doctors that appear to give them little face to face time and appear to be even less concerned with curing them.

As a school psychologist my interest in alternative medicine grew as I searched for alternatives to psychotropic drugs my students were on. Too often I have witnessed active healthy students become "managed" with drugs for their behavior, and left lethargic, lifeless, with a host of side effects they had to contend with. Parents and teachers looking for quick fixes to students' poor behavior and lack of academic motivation lobby physicians to put them on medication for their "disorders" believing that the medications they prescribe will only help.

This book is entitled Holistic *Mental Health* and I believe I have conducted extensive research on traditional treatment as well as alternative treatments for various mental disorders. The disorders I have included are both psychological and physiological because I believe there is a fine line separating the two. Anxiety is usually considered psychosomatic, however, in my experience talking to patients symptoms can certainly be physical; racing pulse, shortness of breath, sweating and even fainting. Headaches and migraines are considered biological in origin usually, but chronic conditions can lead to a very depressive outlook in life.

The recommendations and the treatments discussed for mental disorders in this book treat all disorders primarily in the physical context. Traditional treatment for mental disorders treats symptoms with prescription medications and the treatments are outlined in this book. However, it is accepted in the psychiatric profession that when medication is combined with counseling therapy, results are greatly improved.

The holistic therapies included in this book also treat disorders primarily by addressing physical origins of the disorders, and they may also address the disorder's symptoms. Whether psychiatry or psychological counseling is needed or is beneficial at all in helping mental disorders is not a subject that I discuss in this book. I would encourage readers to investigate that topic further by reading *Psychiatry The Ultimate Betrayal,* by Bruce Wiseman or *The Myth of Mental Illness,* by Thomas Szasz (see suggested further reading) to gain more information on the subject.

My research has in fact given me viable options for mental disorder treatment. The suggestions I make are supported by current research and clinical trials, just like the pharmaceutical company's. These suggestions (see disclaimer) are also backed by hundreds (even thousands) of years of use. The alternative approach to treatment is often more involved than traditional treatment (just take a pill), but, I have come to believe the benefits are extraordinary. Holistic and alternative treatment can cure the disorder, while treating it without harmful side-effects, unlike medications.

~ Dave DiSano, Ph.D.
July, 2005

Preface to the *Revised* Edition

After completion of ***Holistic Mental Health*** in 2005 I realized I should start on a revised edition. As with most technical manuals, information needs to be continually updated. New drugs are continually entering the market, new therapies are continually being tested and new research is continually in the media. And, being primarily a technical manual, ***Holistic Mental Health***, needed to be revised along those lines. In this revision new medications are discussed and entered in the chapters and data tables, and new alternative therapies are discussed for each disorder.

I had however, no idea the additional information I would be exposed to in the past few years pertaining to mental health issues. My life has since taken a whole new direction. That of a "spiritual awakening" through association. As I discussed above, my background was scientific. I approached psychology through biochemistry. My interest in alternative therapies was always bio-chemically based. Just as medications change brain chemistry to alter moods, I investigated and promoted alternative therapies to do the same by "righting" what was wrong or missing in the body. This is the basis for most eastern medicine and treatments.

I also explored and used hypnotherapy, again relying on scientific principles that justified its success. Hypnotherapy simply works through continued re-enforcement. I would work with the patient's subconscious to facilitate something they wanted to change on a conscious level. There was nothing mystical about it. My therapy simply relied on helping people do what they wanted to do by having them listen to positive suggestions daily (via tape or CD). The result was that they changed their thinking and reactions to life, promoting positive changes in their life.

But in the past few years I have come into worlds I've never dreamed I would be directly involved in. Worlds that have little scientific or "clinical" proof, but centuries of documented validation. This is the spiritual realm. The realm science cannot "prove." The realm science continually tries to disprove. Yet it's the realm we all believe in. Some believe in only life after death as in our soul going to heaven when we die (or its alternative). Some believe in, and talk to their guardian angels daily. Some may simply believe in the currency they use that states *"In God We Trust."*

But, do we all not function in both worlds? The explained and the unexplained. One of modern conveniences, of high tech communications and entertainment. One of taking a pill for immediate relief. One in believing in science and technology and all its amazing effects on our everyday life. And one in believing in our scientists and doctors and everything they say without question. However, when we go to them to explain something that they can't see, or test, or explain they are quick to dismiss us, give us a pill, or even commit us to a hospital. And these same scientists and doctors will go to their church and place of worship and pray to something they can't see or explain just like the rest of us.

The unexplained world, that of the unseen, the spirit, the soul, the one I had been fascinated with all my life, was the one I was drawn into in the past few years. This is the world of seers, fortune tellers, mystics, lightworkers, and energy healers. What is called *New Age*, which is occupying larger and larger shelf space in bookstores. But what I have come to experienced was not by reading books. It was through meeting seers, fortune tellers, mystics, and lightworkers. It was through experiencing healing energies, supernatural events and unexplainable coincidences. The *New Age* books verified what I and my wife had been going through, and that others have had similar and even greater experiences.

In the last chapter, *Spiritual Healing*, in this revised edition, I discuss, reference and try to document what traditional science would call that which can not be documented.

Dave DiSano, Ph.D.
February, 2009

Table of Contents

*"If the only tool you have is a hammer,
everything looks like a nail."*

~ **Abraham Maslow**

CHAPTER I:
TRADITIONAL vs. ALTERNATIVE TREATMENT for MENTAL DISORDERS

Healthcare treatment in the U.S. is becoming increasingly controversial, and the public appears to be caught in the middle. However, the public is slowly being educated to alternatives to traditional western *allopathic* medicine, but traditional medicine continually dismisses alternative treatment as quackery. Where is the truth? Is alternative medicine unproven and possibly dangerous? Are there harmful effects when taking non-prescription medicine for illness? If so, why is the news continually filled with FDA warnings of harmful effects of prescription medications, wrongful death law suits against pharmaceutical companies, and bannings and withdrawals of drugs from the market? Which is more harmful? And what kind of treatment is the most effective?

Allopathic treatment promotes the use of prescription medication as a cure for every illness known to man (or woman). Pharmaceutical companies and allopathic physicians continue to promote their drug treatments by aggressive marketing campaigns. It is hard to avoid ads for blood pressure medications, cholesterol, anxiety or depression medications. Television, radio and magazines are filled with ads for medications for mental disorders such as Adderall, Prozac, Paxil, Xanax, or Zoloft. The national evening news appears to be totally "sponsored" by the pharmaceutical companies. Occasionally they do air stories about adverse drug effects, or individual deaths linked to prescription medications. Yet there is evidence the public is not completely satisfied with allopathic methods. Today 40 percent of Americans turn to some sort of nontraditional therapy for what ails them, and they spend about $20 billion a year on these choices [1].

1

This book attempts to answer the above questions with information supported by research and clinical trials for both allopathic medicine and naturopathic treatments for mental disorders.

Mental Illness is on the Rise!

According to the Surgeon General's report on Mental Health, released in December, 1999, David Satcher states that 1 in 5 Americans are affected by mental disorders[2] The World Health Organization's (WHO) 2001, *World Health Report, Mental Health: New Understanding, New Hope* states that mental disorders are among the leading cause of ill health and disability, affecting 450 million people worldwide. Its findings show that mental and behavioral disorders affect 1 in 4 people worldwide[3].

It is often difficult to find a family that may not have, or know of a child that does not have ADHD, an adolescent that is not affected by anxiety or depression an adult that does not get headaches or migraines, or a senior citizen that does not show signs of Alzheimer's Disease.

Alzheimer's Disease is the most common form of dementia with an estimated 5 million people in the United States, and 15 million worldwide affected with the disorder[4]. As the population ages it is estimated that 40 percent of nursing home patients have Alzheimer's Disease and 90 percent have some loss of intellectual function commonly called dementia[5].

Anxiety disorders are among the most common psychiatric disorders in children and foreshadow psychiatric illness later in life. When experienced during childhood, later psychiatric disorders are increased by a factor of 2 to 5 times the risk of mental disorders later in life such as anxiety disorder, major depression, suicide attempts, and hospitalization for psychiatric illness[6]. Adolescents with anxiety disorders are more likely to self-medicate, have an increased risk for failure in school, low paying jobs, and later financial dependence in life. Individuals with anxiety disorders such as social phobia or generalized anxiety disorder have a lifetime risk of 70 percent of developing major depression and increases the likelihood of a suicide attempt by 2 to 6 times[7].

Research indicates 17.5 million American adults, or 1 in 10, will experience depression in their lifetime. Depression results in a 1.8 fold increased risk for physical disability, and a 23 fold increased risk for social disability[8]. Researchers have found that among children 12 years and younger between 1 and 2 percent are depressed. Eight percent of adolescent boys and 10 percent of adolescent girls are depressed. By the end of adolescence more than twice as many girls than boys are depressed[9].

Attention Deficit/ Hyperactivity Disorder (ADHD) is considered the most common childhood neurobehavioral disorder of school-aged children today. Children with ADHD display problematic behaviors at home and 80 percent are believed to display academic performance problems[10]. It is estimated that close to 5 million children today are diagnosed with ADHD[11].

It is estimated that 80 million Americans experience headaches and 50 million have experienced a migraine, with 28 million experiencing frequent migraine attacks[12]. Woman get migraines more than men, as 70 percent of migraine suffers are woman. Thirty percent of migraine suffers get their first attack before age 10, and the disorder is very prevalent among adolescents and young adults. Over $20 billion a year is spent by suffers of headaches and migraines looking for relief [13]. Migraine prevalence is increasing, as evidence is showing an increase of 56 percent in woman and 34 percent in men from 1979 to 1989[14].

Today the criteria for all mental disorders is established by the *Diagnostic and Statistical Manual of Mental Disorders,* published by the American Psychiatric Association. This directory that is a little over 50 years old was first published in 1952. The first issue established diagnostic criteria for 100 mental disorders. The latest edition, *Diagnostic and Statistical Manual of Mental Disorders, 4th Edition-Text Revision (DSM-IV-TR, 2000)* now defines over 300 mental disorders that are recognized by mental health professionals and insurance companies.

The intent of the DSM was to establish reliability in medical diagnosis for mental disorders that was significantly lacking prior to its publication. This was due to the high subjectivity in the diagnosis of mental disorders and the lack of consistent criteria by mental health professionals for the disorders. The DSM appears to have certainly set the norm making the criteria uniform for mental disorders (it is usually considered not to be a disorder if it is not listed in the DSM).

However, reliability studies in the 1990's report that there has been little substantial improvement in the reliability of diagnosis among professionals. It was observed that clinicians will usually gravitate to diagnosis they are comfortable with and it was often observed that they would come up with different diagnosis when presented with the same patient with the same symptoms. The studies also stated that diagnosis can become a self-fulfilling prophecies, for example a child diagnosed with ADHD would consider themselves as broken or limited, and then they act accordingly [15]. In my practice I have seen over the years waves of popular diagnosis prevail. In the 80's and 90's every other child seemed to have a diagnosis of ADHD, now they all appear to have bipolar disorder.

3

Traditional Treatment:

Treatment for mental disorders in the United States usually follows an allopathic format. There is an evaluation by a physician of the symptoms and medication is prescribed. In follow-up visits symptoms and side effects of the medication are discussed and additional medication is prescribed. This pattern continues until the symptoms subside, and if they do not, medication continues seemingly with no end in sight.

Allopathic treatment for Alzheimer's Disease (AD) usually prescribes one of several new treatments for the disease designed to increase the supply of the neurotransmitter, acetycholine. Medications such as physostigmine, tacrine, donepezil, metrifonate, rivastigmine and eptastigmine all have shown to slightly improve AD patient's memories by 3 to 5 percent, however, patients have experienced side effects of nausea, vomiting, dizziness, diarrhea, insomnia, dyspepsia, anorexia, and leg cramps in the clinical trials[16].

Anxiety disorders are treated with anti-anxiety agents, antihistamines, antidepressants, and sedative-hypnotics. Side effects range from ataxia and amnesia, to dry mouth, nausea, convulsions, seizures, and strokes[17].

Medications for depression include tricyclic antidepressants, monoamine oxidase inhibitors, selective serotonin reuptake inhibitors and atypical antidepressants. Side effects of antidepressants can be mild (dry mouth, nausea, headaches) to severe (internal bleeding, coma and death)[18].

Attention Deficit /Hyperactivity Disorder is treated with psycho-stimulate medications and they can carry a wide range of side effects based on the type, dosage and duration of use. Like prescription medications for other mental disorders psycho-stimulates can have mild side effects to severe (high blood pressure, liver damage, Tourette's syndrome, psychosis or drug dependence)[19].

Over-the-counter OTC, medications are usually effective for occasional headaches, however, continual use can lead to drug rebound effects that even create headaches. Allopathic treatment for migraines involves prescribing abortive drugs that stop migraines in progress, and prophylactic drugs that prevent future migraines from striking. Side effects of abortive drugs could include insomnia, anxiety, and agitation. Side effects of prophylatic drugs may include dry mouth, constipation, insomnia, anxiety, high blood pressure, liver damage, and sexual dysfunction[20].

Naturopathic Treatment:

Naturopathic treatment for mental disorders, or alternative medicine, involves therapies such as, nutritional invention, herbal therapy, homeopathy, aromatherapy and relaxation therapies. Research indicates mental disorder like anxiety, depression, ADHD, and migraines may be the result of vitamin or mineral deficiencies. Specific herbs have treated Alzheimer's disease, anxiety, depression, schizophrenia, headaches, and migraines successfully. Aromatherapy has been used to relieve anxiety, depression, headaches and migraines. And relaxation therapies such as meditation, yoga, biofeedback training, and massage therapy have been effective for ADHD, anxiety, depression, headaches, and migraines. These therapies have reported few significant side effects when used correctly, however, misuse of the therapies may occur due to the fact that they are more unregulated in their use than prescription medications [21, 22, 23, 24, 25 , 26].

Medical treatment involving natural substances has been recorded dating back thousands of years. The Chinese document the use of ginkgo for memory loss with the elderly 5,000 years ago. They also record the use of ginseng in the first herb classification texts 3,800 years ago. St. John's wort is believed to have been used for more than 2,000 years for nervous disorders, documented by the Greeks and Romans. The English reported using feverfew, a herbal cure for headaches in the 1640's. European herbal medicine reports the use of sage for memory loss in the 1500's. Kava use for anxiety and stress disorders dates back hundreds of years in the South Pacific [27, 28, 29, 30].

Before the development of prescription medications during the pharmaceutical age of the 20th century, cures in the United States where of course, very natural. The *New American Family Physician,* first published in 1883, lists a number of natural cures as everyday treatments in the 1800s, that are being "rediscovered" today. Their list of medicines includes aloe, chamomile, dandelion, feverfew, foxglove, sassafras, St. John's wort, skullcap and valerian. They also list minerals for specific health conditions such as iron, magnesium and potassium[31].

The use of vitamins to cure illness had a quick rise and fall in the early 1900's. Vitamins, essentially discovered in the first half of the 20th century, became available in pure form between 1935 and 1945. They had a number of positive reports in studies in treating different diseases, however interest in vitamins greatly decreased when sulfa drugs and antibiotics where developed. It appears the majority of physicians in the U.S. jumped on the cure-all-illnesses-with-drugs bandwagon during the mid 1900's. However, a number of researchers such as Linus Pauling, considered the "father of biochemistry" promoted *orthomolecular* medicine, the science and art of healing with nutritional therapy. He was one of the first to promote mega-vitamin therapy (many times greater than RDA's), he is best known for his book *Vitamin C and the Common Cold* (1971), promoting the use of supplements like vitamin C, to cure illness (he is also known for being the only person in history to have won two, unshared, Nobel Prizes) [32]. Researchers at the Mayo Clinic believe that 48 percent of all adult Americans today, take some kind of vitamin or mineral supplement daily[33].

Today alternative therapies appear to be making its way into the allopathic community in the U.S. Medical schools are teaching alternative medicine courses such as therapeutic touch, hospitals and health maintenance organizations offer it and laws in some states require plans to cover it. When combining traditional western allopathic practices with alternative therapies the practice is often called complementary medicine or integrative medicine. Alternative medicine constitutes a huge and rapidly growing industry that major pharmaceutical companies are now participating in[34].

Herbs, vitamins and minerals are considered supplements, and are not regulated like prescription medications or over-the-counter (OTC) products. The 1994 Dietary Supplement Health and Education Act (DSHEA) created a new class of non-prescription products known as "dietary supplements". This legislation defined dietary supplements as a class of products that includes vitamins, minerals, herbs, botanicals, amino acids and other plant derived substances, that are intended for ingestion as a pill, capsule, tablet, or liquid form.

The DSHEA does not allow the Food and Drug Administration (FDA) to authorize or test dietary supplements, and it does not require manufacturers to give the FDA clinical data proving the safety or effectiveness of the supplement. Under the DSHEA a supplement cannot claim to cure or treat a specific medical condition, but may make general statements like "supports mental health", or "boosts stamina and performance." The label must state: "This statement has not been evaluated by the Food and Drug Administration. This product is not intended to diagnose, treat, cure, or prevent any disease." The DSHEA does allow the FDA to restrict or remove a supplement from the market when it can definitively prove harm[35].

Safety of Naturopathic Medicine:

The FDA began to evaluate the safety and efficacy of nonprescription OTC drugs in 1972. They place their findings in one of three categories: Category I, *Safe and Effective*, Category II, *Unsafe and/or Ineffective*, or Category III, *Insufficient Evidence to Decide*. The FDA evaluation panels do not conduct research, they only review studies submitted to them, usually by pharmaceutical companies. By 1990 the FDA had rendered judgments on 258 drug ingredients, and few herbs on that list made Category I. If there was not enough information submitted the herb, or supplement was automatically placed in either Category II or III. It usually takes a number of expensive studies to determine if a herb works and is safe.

Since herbs, vitamins and minerals can not be patented, there is no financial incentive for a manufacturer to invest hundreds of thousands of dollars to study something other manufacturers can easily imitate without cost. So without the research, most herbs and supplements were classified as unsafe/ineffective or unproven by default. However, this does not mean a supplement is not ineffective or unsafe just because it has not met with FDA approval.

For example, the FDA did not approve prune juice due to lack of evidence, yet it has been universally recognized as an effective laxative, and the same was true for eucalyptus oil, found in many cough preparations, which was declared unsafe and ineffective as a cough remedy. The most popular selling herbs, St. John's wort, ginkgo, ginseng, Echinacea and garlic have not been evaluated by the FDA, or approved, yet they have been used for thousands of years as safe and effective remedies[36].

Most drugs are approved by the FDA after 6 months of study. The submitted studies may in fact take longer by the pharmaceuticals. Yet, the long-term safety of the drug unfortunately is tested by the public. Many complications and drug side-effects do not show up during the drug trials, and certainly are not present when people start mixing other prescriptions with the new ones they are taking. Physicians try to monitor these drug interactions, but sometimes they are too late when a fatal combination is observed. Such was the case with prescription arthritis pain medication, when the long-term observations, often after 18 months of use, indicated higher incidences of heart attacks and strokes among uses. Or an ADHD drug that was taken off the market due to increased incidence of heart attacks and strokes in children.

In comparing safety records of alternative supplements to prescription medications some startling facts surface. Mainstream media fueled by allopathic physicians regularly warns against the dangers of "unproven" supplements and herbal remedies. But what is the reported number of people who have died using herbs and supplements?

According to the FDA, between 1993 and 1998, federal, state and local agencies reported 184 deaths by people taking non-prescription supplements. Most of these deaths were associated with weight loss formulas. Compare that number to the reported number of people who die in hospitals every year of the side effects of properly prescribed pharmaceutical drugs: more than 100,000, every year. Add to that number, another 100,000 who die every year due to "medical errors" (some health experts estimate as many as 250,000 deaths per year). Deaths from pharmaceuticals comprise the fourth leading cause of death, right behind heart disease, cancer, and stroke.

In addition to those that die in hospitals, *The Journal of the American Medical Association (JAMA),* reports an estimated 2 million more people require hospitalization every year due to adverse side effects from prescription medications, out of a possible 3.6 million drug misadventures per year[36]. These facts appear to go unreported by the news media, perhaps due to the $250 billion per year pharmaceutical industry, and the $30 billion the pharmaceutical companies spend each year in advertising with the media. It appears that "alternative" remedies have quite a better safety record than prescription medications.

CHAPTER II:
Alzheimer's DISEASE

Alzheimer's Disease (AD) is the most common form of dementia with an estimated 5 million individuals in the United States, and 15 million people worldwide currently are afflicted with the disease. AD was first discovered in 1906 by Alois Alzheimer, who observed unusual changes in the brain of a woman who died at age 55, five years after developing dementia. Using special silver stains to more clearly reveal the structure of this woman's brain cells, he discovered that the cerebral cortex contained abnormal nerve cells with tangled fibers and clusters of degenerating nerve endings. It is this development of abnormal plaques and tangled neurons in the cerebral cortex that characterizes AD.

The *Diagnostic and Statistical Manual of Mental Disorders, 4th Edition-Text Revision (DSM-IV-TR, 2000)* lists AD as one of several dementia disorders. Its prevalence increases dramatically with age, rising from 6 percent in males and 8 percent in females at age 65, to 11 percent in males and 14 percent in females at age 85. By age 90 the prevalence rate rises to 21 percent in males and 25 percent in females, and by age 95 it is 36 percent in males and 41 percent in females [1, 2, 3, 4]

Types of Alzheimer's Disease:

The *DSM-IV-TR* classifies AD as two main subtypes: AD with Early Onset, and AD with Late Onset. Early onset AD is dementia with onset before age

65, and late onset is AD dementia after age 65. With these subtypes there are also two coded subtypes used: .10 Without Behavioral Disturbance, if no clinically significant behavioral disturbance is present, and, .11 With Behavioral Disturbance, if there is behavioral disturbance present (e.g. wandering, agitation). The diagnostic criteria for the AD dementia is based on:

A. The development of multiple cognitive deficits manifested by both:

1. Memory impairment (impaired ability to learn new information or to recall previously learned information).
2. One (or more) of the following cognitive disturbances:
   a. aphasia (language disturbance).
   b. apraxia (impaired ability to carry out motor activities despite in tact motor function).
   c. agnosia (failure to recognize or identify objects despite intact sensory function).
   d. disturbance in executive functioning (i.e., planning, organizing, sequencing, abstracting).

B. The cognitive deficits in Criteria A1 and A2 (above) each cause significant impairment in social or occupational functioning and represent a significant decline from a previous level of functioning.

C. The course is characterized by gradual onset and continuing cognitive decline.

D. The cognitive deficits in Criteria A1 and A2 are not due to any of the following:
1. Other central nervous system conditions that cause progressive deficits in memory and cognition (e.g., cerebrovascular disease, Parkinson's disease, Huntington's disease, subdural hematoma, normal-pressure hydrocephalus, brain tumor).
2. Systemic conditions that are known to cause dementia (e.g., hypothyroidism, vitamin B12 or folic acid deficiency, niacin deficiency, hypercalcemia, neurosyphilis, HIV infection).
3. Substance-induced conditions.

E. The deficits do not occur exclusively during the course of a delirium.

F.   The disturbance is not better accounted for by another Axis I
disorder (e.g., Major Depressive Disorder, Schizophrenia).

Stages of Alzheimer's Disease

The *DSM-IV-TR* states that diagnosis of AD can be made only when other
etiologies for the dementia have been ruled out due to the difficulty of obtaining
direct pathological evidence of the presence of AD. In the majority of cases,
brain atrophy is present in dementia of the Alzheimer's type, with wider cortical
sulci and larger cerebral ventricles than would be expected given the normal
aging process. This may be demonstrated by computed tomography (CT) or
magnetic resonance imaging (MRI). Microscopic examination usually reveals
histopathological changes, including senile plagues, neurofribrillary tangles,
granulovascular degeneration, neuronal loss, astrocytic gliosis, and amyloid
angiopathy. Lewy bodies are sometimes seen in the cortical neurons[5].

Individuals who develop AD progress, usually slowly, through various
stages. There is a clinical loss of 3 to 4 points per year on standard assessment
instruments such as the Mini-Mental State Exam. It often begins with general
forgetfulness of recent events or recently acquired information, such as people's
names or where something was put.

In a second stage of AD, the individual's confusion is more noticeable.
They mix up their words, their speech is often aimless and repetitious, and
there are visible deficits in their concentration and short-term memory
(aphasia, apraxia, and agnosia).

When an individual progresses to the third stage of AD they are no
longer able to manage their daily basic needs. Individuals develop gait and
motor disturbances. They may forget to eat, or dress properly, they may create
hazards at home by leaving a stove or iron on, or may get lost in their own
neighborhoods.

In the fourth stage of AD the individual is no longer able to take care of
themselves, they are unable to communicate or recognize immediate family
members, they eventually become mute and bedridden. The average duration
of the illness from onset of the symptoms to death is 8 to 10 years [6,7].

Early Identification of Alzheimer's Disease:

Although the progression of the disease is usually evident in the diagnosis of
AD, the characteristic plaques of AD can only be identified in an autopsy.
However, researchers in France have developed an automated system for
measuring brain tissue loss using magnetic resonance imaging (MRI)

technology. In AD the buildup of plaques leads to brain cell and tissue death. And the most damage occurs in the hippocampus, which affects memory.

The automated MRI system helps in diagnosing AD by speeding up the process of visually measuring shrinkage in the hippocampus consistent with the development of AD. More accurate diagnosis of AD can lead to earlier treatment of the disease [8].

Causes of Alzheimer's Disease:

Environmental Causes:

Carl Pfeiffer in *Nutrition and Mental Illness,* [9] suggests two possible causes for the entanglement of nerve fibers found in the brains of AD individual's. He believes that continued involuntary consumption of aluminum contributes to the development of these plaques responsible for AD or, possibly that diseases like arteriosclerosis and atherosclerosis cause decreased blood flow to the brain and nerve cells. This decreased blood flow in turn causes a decreased oxygen supply in the brain that leads to the senility of AD.

Louise Tenney, author of *Nutritional Guide: A Comprehensive Reference for Better Health,* suggests that either high aluminum concentrations in the brain or the reduced activity of the neurotransmitter acetylcholine, responsible for message transmission between nerve cells, as possible causes of AD [10]. Recent research indicates that aluminum increases the formation of advanced glycosylation end products (AGE) which are proteins that accumulate in the brain as a result of toxins. AGE proteins induce inflammation in the brain and increase oxidative stress in brain cells, causing their early destruction. It is believed that aluminum is a neurotoxin that can impair cognition and has been found to interfere with more than 50 neurochemical reactions. For many years scientists have observed that the individuals who are exposed to high levels of soluble aluminum through their water supply, aluminum cookware, or medications like aluminum containing antacids, have an increased risk of developing AD[11,12].

A study by Elisabeth Koss, Ph.D., of *Case Western Reserve University* reported that high levels of lead exposure have been shown to increase the likelihood by 3.4 times of developing AD. In the study, occupational histories of 185 people with AD was compared to 303 people without the disease. In addition to lead, researchers examined exposure to aluminum, copper, iron, mercury, zinc, and solvents such as paint thinners, and cleaning fluids. Only prolonged exposure to lead was found to increase the risk of developing AD[13].

Zinc has also been linked to AD in controversial ways. Some scientists suggest that too little zinc is at fault, while others believe too much zinc can contribute to neuron death by causing soluble beta-amyloid, from the cerebrospinal fluid, to form clumps similar to Alzheimer's plaques in the brain. There are a number of studies that link a zinc deficiency with the symptoms of Alzheimer's[14].

Genetic Causes:

Recent theories suggest that the plaques in the brain's of AD individuals are composed of protein fragments of beta-amyloid. The beta-amyloid plaques kill or damage brain cells producing memory loss and other AD symptoms. The brain makes beta-amyloid by chopping up a larger molecule, amyloid precursor protein (APP), with enzymes called beta-secretases. The discovery that the gene identified that carries beta-secretases is on chromosome 21 has increased interest in this theory. It has been observed that individuals with Down syndrome, who have three copies of chromosome 21, usually develop AD if they live long enough. Late onset AD is believed to have genetic components. AD in some families has been shown to be inherited as an autosomal dominant trait with linkage to several chromosomes, including chromosome 1, 14, and 21[15,16].

A study reported in *The New England Journal of Medicine,* found a link between individuals that are homozygous for the ∈4 allele for apolipoprotein E have reduced glucose metabolism in the same regions of the brain as patients with AD (also known as ApoE4). This suggests evidence that the presence of the ∈4 allele (specific gene) is a risk factor for AD. It is believed the defective gene causes ineffective synthesis of cell membranes responsible for protecting the brain's neurons from injury. This causes the immune system to respond with an overproduction of interleukin-6 that stimulates beta-amyloid (a protein) to break off from its parent molecule, amyloid precursor protein (APP). Beta- amyloid causes free radical injury to cells promoting neuron death in the area responsible for producing acetylcholine, a neurotransmitter responsible for memory and cognition[17,18,19].

Scientists from the Feinstein Institute for Medical Research in Manhasset, NY report finding a new genetic risk factor for AD. They have identified a gene called CALHM1 that increases the likelihood of the occurrence of late onset AD (AD occurring age 65 or older). This gene is linked to a calcium channel that can increase the production of amyloid proteins in brain cells that create the amyloid plaques believed to cause AD. Having one or more alleles of CALHM1 can increase the risk factor of AD from 44 to 77%. Their research states that there may be 20 genes, or 20 or so risk factors for increasing the risk of developing AD, but that ApoE4 and CALHM1 are the most robust factors identified to this point [20].

Allopathic Treatment:

Treatment for Alzheimer's Disease appears to be taking two distinct avenues. The first addressing the possible biochemical abnormalities that may be causing the disorder and treating AD through the development of new drugs or using traditional allopathic treatment. The second, by using what has been lacking in an individual's diet, or the use of supplements that may contradict environmental toxins, which can be called naturopathic treatment to prevent or delay AD.

Estrogen replacement therapy, or hormone replacement therapy (HRT), was initially thought to be a possible treatment to prevent or slow down the symptoms of AD. Several epidemiological studies suggested that women on estrogen replacement get AD less frequently and at a later age. However, recent findings suggest it is not as an effective as a treatment for women who already have AD.

In a study of 42 women with mild to moderate dementia randomized to receive estrogen or a placebo, researchers at the *University of Southern California School of Medicine,* Los Angeles, CA found no significant difference in mood or cognitive ability between treatment and control groups.

Recent studies published in the *Journal of the American Medical Association* and the *Journal of the National Cancer Institute,* report the use of estrogen increases woman's risk of breast cancer. Short-term side effects of HRT includes irregular bleeding, fluid retention, breast tenderness, and headaches. Other long-term effects could include uterine cancer, heart problems, higher triglyceride levels, gallbladder disease, and increased blood clotting [21, 22].

Drugs Approved for Treatment of Alzheimer's Disease:

Two classes of drugs are now FDA approved for the treatment of AD: Cholinesterase inhibitors (Antilirium, Aricept, Cognex, Exelon, and Razadyne) and memantime (Namenda), that regulates a neurotransmitter called glutamate.

The cholinesterase inhibitors increase the supply of the neurotransmitter, acetycholine, a loss of which is thought to bring on AD. Among the drugs available today are physostigmine (Antilirium), tacrine (Cognex), donepezil

(Aricept), galantamine (Razadyne or Reminyl), eptastigmine, and rivastigmine (Exelon). Physotigmine, tacrine, donepezil, and eptasigmine are reversible inhibitors that bind to acetylcholinesterase, inhibiting the formation of the enzyme acetylcholine complex. Rivastigmine does not directly inhibit the formation of the enzyme acetylcholine, but decreases the enzyme activity directly.

Memantime (Namenda) may improve memory awareness and the ability to perform daily functions by blocking the action of a protein glutamate. A 2008 study reported that when memantime is combined with a cholinesterase inhibitor memory loss and functional declines are slowed even more than when one drug is used alone.

All of these medications have shown small improvement in cognitive functioning as measured by scores on Alzheimer's Disease Assessment Scale (3 to 5 percent). However, the adverse effects associated with the drugs are considerable. The most common side effects were nausea (up to 79 percent with physostigmine, 35 percent with rivastigmine), vomiting (57 percent with physostigmine), dizziness (30 percent with physostigmine), diarrhea (26 percent with physostigmine), insomnia (14 percent with donepezil), other side effects included dyspepsia, anorexia, and leg cramps. In trials of rivastigmine up to 43 percent of the patients withdrew due to adverse effects . Memantime's side effects could include confusion, constipation, coughing, dizziness, hallucinations, headache, high blood pressure, pain, and insomnia [23, 24].

A drug that preserves acetylcholine, galantamine, has been shown to improve the functioning of AD patients. Acetylcholine is a brain chemical vital for nerve cells to communicate with each other. In a study of 353 AD patients treated with galantamine, it was reported they had maintained or improved their scores on a an assessment test one year later. Galantamine has been approved for use in Sweden and is being considered for approval in the U.S. [25]. Three other drugs currently approved by the FDA, Exelon (Rivastigmine), Aricept (Donepezil), and Cognex (Tacrine), all inhibit the breakdown of acetylcholine [26, 27].

Anti-inflammatory drugs are believed to play a role in slowing the cognitive decline of AD. Inflammation is thought to be closely associated with the accumulation of beta amyloid plaque. Deposition of amyloid appears to incite an inflammatory response that releases cytokines, which kills neurons. Anti-inflammatory drugs such as Naproxen and Dapsone are currently undergoing clinical trials to test their effect on AD patients [28] [29].

A different type of drug treatment is still in the development stage. Researchers are planning trials on an AD vaccine. The vaccine prompts the immune system to destroy protein that forms destructive plaque in the brain of AD patients. In animal tests it prevented plaque formation in young mice and reversed plaque buildup in older mice [30].

The only drugs approved for AD at this time in the U.S. are donepezil (Aricept), rivastigmine (Exelon), tacrine (Cognex), and memantime (Namenda) [31]. AD and dementia patients should not take antipsychotic drugs. A FDA news release in 2005, warned physicians that may give patients with dementia antipsychotic drugs to control their delusions and hallucinations reported that that such drugs increase the risk of death [32].

Table 2-1
Summary of Allopathic Treatment for Alzheimer's Disease [23, 27, 40] :

Drug: (Brand name)	*Acting mechanism:*	*Possible side effects:*
HRT (Hormone Replacement Therapy)	Increased hormones; estrogen	Irregular bleeding, fluid retention, breast tenderness, headaches. Long-term use: cancer, heart problems gallbladder disease, blood clots.
Physotigmine (Antilirium)	Increases acetylcholine by acting as a reverse Inhibitor.	Nausea, vomiting, dizziness, diarrhea.
Tacrine (Cognex)	Increases acetylcholine by acting as a reverse Inhibitor.	Nausea, dizziness, diarrhea.
Donepezil (Aricept)	Increases acetylcholine by acting as a reverse Inhibitor.	Insomnia, nausea, vomiting, diarrhea.
Rivastigmine (Exelon)	Decreases enzyme activity.	Nausea, dizziness, leg cramps.
Eptastigmine	Increases acetylcholine by acting as a reverse Inhibitor.	Nausea, dizziness.
Galantamine (Reminyl)	Preserves acetylcholine.	Nausea, vomiting, diarrhea.

Naproxen (Naprosen)	Anti-inflammatory action slows the accumulation of beta-amyloid plaque.	Rash, hives, dizziness, headache, diarrhea, stomach cramps.
Dapsone (Aviosulfon)	Anti-inflammatory action slows the accumulation of beta-amyloid plaque.	Rash, abdominal pain, dizziness, blurred vision, anemia, headache, itching, vomiting.

Naturopathic Therapy:

Naturopathic Therapy for Alzheimer's Disease involves the use of supplements such as vitamins, minerals or herbs, and recommends activity. This type of treatment is often considered more preventative by the medical community, as it is thought to slow down the onset or the progression of AD rather than cure the disease. However, allopathic treatment does the same. Current drugs for AD will only slow the progression of the disease, not cure it.

Ginkgo

The most highly publicized natural treatment for AD has been with the use of **ginkgo** (*Ginkgo biloba*). Ginkgo is one of the oldest living tree species, dating back over 200 million years. Originally found in eastern Asia and China after the Ice Age, today it flourishes throughout North America, Europe and Asia. The ginkgo tree is a dioecous species, meaning it has both male and female variants. The tree can grow to 125 feet tall and live 1,000 years.

The Chinese documented the positive effects of ginkgo 5,000 years ago, where ancient Chinese herbal medical text noted that ginkgo leaves could reverse memory loss in the elderly and ease breathing problems. Not until the 18th century did the West the "discover" ginkgo. A German physician and botanist encountered the tree on a trip to Japan, where he recorded its medicinal uses in his writings. The tree was first brought to Europe in 1730, where it was planted in Holland. By the 19th century it was found throughout Europe, and first brought to America soon after the Revolutionary War.

Since the 1950s more than 400 papers on Ginkgo, most from German investigators, have appeared in medical literature. Today ginkgo is widely used in Germany and France where it is one of the most common medications prescribed by doctors, and one of the most widely over-the-counter (OTC) medications used without prescriptions in lower doses [33, 34, 35].

More than 50 controlled clinical trials confirm that ginkgo as a viable treatment for diminished memory and concentration, increased absentmindedness, confusion, energy loss, tiredness, depression, dizziness, and tinnitus (ringing in the ears). It is believed to be as effective as prescription medication like tacrine and donepezil, but without the side effects. The herb has been reported to treat dementia, and a recent English study confirmed this contention. In a study, conducted by the *Medical Research Centre* at the *University of Surrey, Guildford, England,* thirty-six healthy volunteers between the ages of 30 and 59 were placed in one of five groups who received various doses of ginkgo biloba extract (GBE) or a placebo. The participants took memory tests before and after taking the herb. Results indicated even a one-time dose of GBE can improve concentration, focus and alertness for younger and older adults as well. The greatest improvement came from participants ages 50 to 59 [36].

The key to ginkgo's mind-sharpening success researchers believe may be a group of active ingredients known as flavoniods, which are antioxidants also found in many fruits and vegetables. Ginkgo formulas usually contain 24 percent flavonoids, along with terpene lactones, also found in ginkgo, seems to keep red blood cells and platelets from forming clots. This increases blood flow and therefore oxygen to the brain boosting mental functioning.

Two recent German studies showed impressive effects of ginkgo after regular use. One study found that ginkgo improved brain function by 72 percent on average after three months of use by 99 percent patients who had suffered brain disturbances for two years. In another study of 200 patients, of an average age of 69, who had memory problems for four years, showed that 71 percent improved after three months of use of ginkgo, compared with 32 percent on placebo.

A comprehensive study review in 1998, found over 50 articles reporting ginkgo's effect on cognitive function and a total of 424 patients meeting clinical scientific study standards. Patients with AD who received 120 to 240 mg per day of standardized ginkgo extract showed significant improvement in cognitive function after 3 to 6 months of use. No significant side effects were reported with use of ginkgo in any of the trials [37, 38, 39, 40, 41].

Ginkgo's main pharmacological agents are thought to be flavone glycosides (isorhamnetin, quercetin, and kaempferol), bioflavonoids, and terpene lactones, that are called ginkgolides. Ginkgo has anti-inflammatory activity that protects diseased arteries from further damage. Evidence suggests that ginkgo's flavone glycosides may be even more effective antioxidants than either vitamin E or beta-carotene. Ginkgo's bioflavonoids help strengthen capillary walls and makes them more resilient to trauma. Ginkgo's ginkgolides discourages blood platelet stickiness, reducing formation of blood clots and plaque buildup. Research from France indicate that ginkgo can restore the ability of brain cells to transmit and receive signals from neurotransmitters that govern brain activity.

The terpene lactones may also play a role in the protection of nerve cells. Ginkgo also increases glucose metabolism in the brain, increasing the brain's "energy". Ginkgo can be taken in tablet form, liquid, and dried leaves for tea. Doses required for therapeutic effect are 120 to 240 mg of standardized extract divided in one to three times per day.

Ginkgo should not be used by individuals on anticoagulants (blood thinners), with bleeding or clotting disorders or serious liver disease, or when pregnant. Rare side effects of ginkgo use includes stomach or intestinal upset, headaches, allergic skin reaction and mild transient dizziness. When taken with SSRIs ginkgo has been reported to reverse the sexual side effects caused by the SSRIs [42, 43, 44, 45].

Ginseng

Ginseng is a herb with reported memory boosting properties. Ginseng was listed in the first Chinese classification of herbs in 1,800 BC as the highest among the "superior" herbs. The most common types of ginseng, Asian ginseng, *Panax ginseng,* and American ginseng, *Panax quinquefolius,* have very different properties.

Asian ginseng is considered a warm stimulating herb, and is used to offset the conditions associated with aging. American ginseng is a cooling, sedating herb, used to reduce stress. Studies with Asian ginseng with both animals and humans report its ability to stimulate the nervous system, improve learning ability, increase mental functioning, and improve memory and recall which may make it a beneficial treatment for AD.

Ginseng can be taken in tea, powdered extract or capsules. Recommended doses are 100 to 250 mg of ginseng containing 4 to 7 percent of ginsenosides (active ingredient) in capsules. Ginseng may cause irritability when consumed with caffeine or other stimulates. Ginseng is not recommended for people on anticoagulant medication such as Warfarin, or Ticlopidine, a platelet inhibiting drug, as it may cause increased bleeding, and there has been a case of hypomania of a woman who took ginseng with Phenelzine (Nardil), a MAOI used for depression [46, 47, 48].

Sage

Another herb reported to have some effect on AD is **sage**, *Salvia officinalis*. Sage has been reported in ancient folklore as a herb with a reputation in improving memory. It has been used in traditional Chinese medicine, Ayurvedic medicine, and European herbal medicine since the 1500's.

A study by Peter J. Houghton, Ph.D., professor of pharmacognosy at King's College in London, England, found that volatile oils in sage contained two constituents that were effective against the development of AD. Alphapinene and 1,8-cineole have distinct activity against an enzyme called acetylcholinesterase, which is believed to be closely associated with the development of AD. It is believed that inhibition of acetylcholinesterase might be helpful in slowing the progression of the disease [49, 50].

Vitamin E

Vitamin E has also been found to significantly benefit patients with AD. An article in *Environmental Nutrition* [51] reports a two year study with 350 men and women with AD who took one of four treatments: Eldepryl (a Parkinson's Disease medication), 2,000 IU's of vitamin E, a combination of the two, or a placebo. The study concluded that individuals who took either Eldepryl or vitamin E had a delay in decline in their mental abilities. The positive effect high doses of vitamin E has on AD has been contrasted to research that shows low levels of vitamin E have been found to be associated with dementia both in older people and in the context of Down's syndrome.

Vitamin E may have a potential therapeutic role in AD by protecting the integrity of the muscarinic receptor (frontal cortex neurons). Antioxidants such as vitamin E appears to have a positive role against the free-radical damage that AD patients appear to be very susceptible to [52].

A report at the 60th annual conference of the American Academy of Neurology (April, 2008) stated that Vitamin E can help AD patients live longer. The report cites a study by Valory Pavlik, PhD, of Baylor's College of Medicine, that involved 847 AD patients who took 2,000 IU's of Vitamin E were 26% less likely to die when viewed 5 years later [53].

In addition to vitamin E, other antioxidants that boost blood flow and energy metabolism that aid in slowing down the onset or the effects of AD are **vitamin C** and **selenium** [54].

Choline

Choline is a member of the vitamin B-complex family and is also a fat emulsifier. It is believed to be one of the few substances able to penetrate the blood-brain barrier, which ordinarily protects the brain against variations in the daily diet.

Choline can go directly into the brain cells to produce a chemical that aids memory, perhaps by emulsifying cholesterol so that it does not settle on artery walls of blood vessels [55]. Chorine is also believed to stimulate the production of acetylcholine, thereby improving one's short-term memory [56].

Phosphatidylserine

Phosphatidylserine (PS) is a fat-soluble phospholipids that exists naturally in the brain. It is responsible for repairing the outside membrane of the brain as it wears out with age. PS supplementation is believed to have positive effects on age-related cognitive decline.

Clinical testing on the supplement convinced the FDA that the PS is safe, and allowed claims that PS may reduce the risk of dementia and cognitive decline in the elderly. PS is found in soybeans and dark-green leafy vegetables. Supplements are derived from cows or soybeans. For memory loss, significant problems with day to day functioning, or early stages of AD, 300 mg of a soy-derived PS is recommended daily [57].

Coenzyme Q10

Coenzyme Q10 is an antioxidant that increases mental alertness. Studies are being conducted on early stage Parkinson's disease, a degenerative disease that causes delays in motor control due to impaired delivery of dopamine in the brain. It is believed that Coenzyme Q10 benefits brain function at doses of 100 to 300 mg per day. If impairment is occurring 1,200 mg daily is recommended [58].

DHA

The UCLA Alzheimer's Disease Research Center reports that people suffering from AD have low levels of a brain protein called LR11 (due to diet or a genetic mutation that reduces LR11). LR11 helps clear the brain of amyloid precursor protein, which is essential for the production of the brain-gumming beta-amyloid plaque that clogs the brain. DHA (docosahexanoic acid), a fish oil fatty acid, causes brain cells to produce LR11, that in turn can help reduce the formation of beta-amyloid plaques [59] .

Curry Spice-Turmeric

Another substance found to reduce the formation of beta-amyloid plaques is a compound found in curry spice, turmeric. A research team from the Medical School at the University of California, found that a compound called bisdemethoxycurcumin in turmeric helps reduce the formation of beta-amyloid plaques [60].

Green Tea

A two year study using green tea by the University of Newcastle in Great Britain found that green tea may delay cognitive decline. The study using 70 year old individuals showed that those consuming more green tea daily had less mental decline then those that consumed less [61].

Huperzine A

Huperzine A is a derivative of the Chinese herb *Huperzia serrata*. It has positive effects in brain metabolism by blocking the enzyme that destroys acetylcholine, a neurotransmitter chemical that plays a key role in short-term memory. A clinical study on its effectiveness with AD patients is currently underway by the National Institute of on Aging using 200 or 400 mcg of Huperzine twice a day [62].

Combination Supplements

Louise Tenney, author of *Nutritional Guide A Comprehensive Reference for Better Health* (1997), believes AD can be prevented, delayed or controlled with a nutritional supplement plan. Tenney recommends the following vitamins: B-complex with extra thiamin (B1), pyridoxine (B6), niacin (B3), C, and E. Minerals such as copper, manganese, magnesium, iodine, silver, sulphur, selenium, potassium, phosphorus and zinc are important for memory and brain function (usually found in a vitamin-mineral supplement). She recommends the following herbs: Alfalfa, burdock, and butcher's broom to improve circulation, chaparral, Echinacea, and garlic to dissolve cholesterol, and ginkgo, ginger, ginseng, gotu kola, rosemary, red clover, skullcap, suma and valerian all increase brain function [63].

A 1996 multicenter study with 450 patients with AD demonstrated significant reduction in their rate of decline when taking **ALC supplements**. ALC is a natural substance derived from the amino acid L-carnitine, and works with L-carnitine to help fatty acids cross into inner mitochondrial membranes.

ALC may help protect against AD by acting as an active antioxidant that protects the cell membranes of neurons against free radical production. ALC appears to be a safe, effective treatment for anyone diagnosed with AD, and recommended doses are 2 grams daily between meals [64].

Cell membranes in the brain also require lipids or fats to function properly. Phosphatidylserine (PS), a fatty acid, helps protect the cell from free radical damage. The omega-3 fatty acid docosahexanoic acid (DHA) acts as a natural calcium channel blocker, helping to prevent beta amyloid from forming. PS is found in soy lecithin extract and DHA is found in fish oils. Cold water fish such as salmon is also an excellent source of DHA. Recommended doses are 300 mg of each in supplements daily [65].

Physical Activity

Exercise is considered the "Fountain of Youth," and for AD it is imperative to remain active. Jytte Lokvig and John Becker in *Alzheimer's A to Z* recommends a number of activities senior citizens can be involved in to stay "young" and active. Caregivers are encouraged to take the lead in helping with activities such as walks, dancing, swimming and even sitting exercises if the individual is not mobile. Games are extremely important for mental stimulation and they recommend card games, checkers, board games, word games, and crossword puzzles. Lawn games like croquet, ring toss, horseshoes or lawn bowling stimulate the body and mind [66].

New Research

Studies that are in preliminary phases, that have been conducted on research animals and not with human trials, that are not "FDA approved" and have yielded promising results include the use of an antihistamine, an epilepsy drug, and a form of B-3.

A study from Russia using Dimebon, a Russian antihistamine, reports when 183 patients with mild to moderate AD were given Dimebon the disease was stabilized for at least 18 months. The drug appears to reduce the levels of beta-amyloid. There is also evidence that it affects cellular mitochondria, the power plants that energize cells, fixing a defect that kills brain cells [67].

Researchers from Canada's University of British Columbia report positive results on mice given Valproic acid, an epilepsy drug. They report that the drug may have benefits before AD becomes severe. Mice in the study did not develop as much brain plaques when given Valproic acid [68].

Nicotinamide, a form of vitamin B-3, may help AD patients retain their memory. A study published in *The Journal of Neuroscience*, (11/5/08) reports research from the University of California where mice were fed dissolved nicotinamide in drinking water. The mice appeared to have improved short-term memory and the nicotinamide prevented mental defects in mice with AD. They believe that the nicotinamide improves the stability of microtubules, the scaffolding within brain cells along which nerve signals travel [69].

TauRX Therapeutics of Singapore is developing a drug called *Remember*, that dissolves tau tangles, that are fibrous tangles found in AD patient's brains. In clinical trials in the U.K. and in Singapore, patients treated with *Remember* had no decline in cognitive function. This is an important study researchers state because tau tangles appear in the brain before AD symptoms appear, and by preventing them AD progression may be arrested [70].

An Australian firm, Prana Biotechnology is developing another plaque-busting drug called PBT2. This drug has been shown to be able to break down beta-amyloid-42. In a clinical trial involving 78 mild AD patients it significantly reduced the beta-amyloid levels. Researchers believe by combing PBT2 with an anti-tau drug like *Remember*, and a drug like Dimebon, significant improvements can be achieve [71].

Table 2-2
Summary of Naturopathic Treatment for Alzheimer's Disease [23, 26, 44] :

Common Name/ (scientific name):	Acting mechanism:	Possible side effects/ Interactions:
Ginkgo *(Ginkgo biloba)*	Increases cerebral blood flow, reduces blood clots, strengthens capillary walls, anti-inflammatory.	Upset stomach, headaches, allergic skin reactions, mild dizziness, Reaction with anticoagulants, should not be taken when pregnant.
Ginseng *(Panax ginseng)*	Stimulates the nervous system, aiding memory and mental functioning.	Irritability when taken with caffeine or stimulates. Reaction with anticoagulants.
Sage *(Salvia officinalis)*	Inhibits acetyl cholinesterase.	Reaction with anticoagulants.
Vitamin E	Antioxidant, protects frontal cortex neurons.	Nausea, vomiting, fatigue. Reaction with anticoagulants.
Vitamin B-3 (Niacin)	Can improve memory by aiding cellular health.	None
Choline	Stimulates the production of acetycholine, emulsifies cholesterol.	None.
ACL *(amino acid L-carnitine)*	Antioxidant, protects neurons against damage, promotes phospholipid metabolism, enhance brain energy.	None.

DHA (*Docosahex- anoic acid*)	Acts as a natural calcium channel blocker, helping to prevent beta amyloid from forming. Increases LH11.	None.

CONCLUSIONS:

As it is with many health problems individuals have a choice of treatment. They can choose traditional "drug" therapy or the non-traditional natural therapy using supplements. The number of available drugs to treat Alzheimer's Disease seems to be overwhelming. However, positive results of the drug treatments are not. Most drugs appear to still be going through trials and are in the development stage. And, it is not clear which drug treatment should be used because they each attack a different cause of AD. Should drugs that increase acetycholine be used, or anti-inflammatory drugs be used, or should a vaccine be used? Most likely treatment would be recommended based on what the physician believes to be the cause of AD.

Current theories on the cause of AD include a biochemical chain reaction of beta-amyloid proteins resulting in causing free radical protection and damage to brain cell neurons. Researchers believe there are genetic links to the apolipoprotein E allele that leads individuals to be more susceptible to the production of beta amyloid.

Environmental toxins such as aluminum, lead, and zinc, may also lead to the development of AD. High levels of these metals have been found in the brains of AD patients. Inadequate nutrients may promote the development of AD by not fighting toxins or free radicals damage, or by giving the neurons the proper nourishment to function properly.

Allopathic treatment uses several medications that have shown to slow the progression of AD. Estrogen replacement therapy, or hormone replacement therapy (HRT), was initially thought to be a possible treatment to prevent or slow down the symptoms of AD. Several studies suggested that women on estrogen replacement get AD less frequently and at a later age. However, recent findings suggest it is not as an effective as a treatment for women who already have AD. Side effects of HRT may include irregular bleeding, fluid retention, breast tenderness, headaches, uterine cancer, heart problems, higher triglyceride levels, gallbladder disease, and increased blood clotting.

Newer drugs for AD such as Physostigmine, Tacrine (*Cognex*), Donepezil

(*Aricept*), Metrifonate, Rivastigmine (*Exelon*), and eptastigmine. increase the supply of the neurotransmitter, acetycholine, a loss of which is thought to bring on AD. Physotigmine, Tacrine, Donepezil, and Eptasigmine are reversible inhibitors that bind to acetylcholinesterase, inhibiting the formation of the enzyme acetylcholine complex. Rivastigmine does not directly inhibit the formation of the enzyme acetylcholine, but decreases the enzyme activity directly. Metrifonate is considered a pseudo irreversible inhibitor of acetylcholinesterase. All of these medications have shown small improvement in cognitive functioning as measured by scores on Alzheimer's Disease Assessment Scale (3 to 5 percent), however, side effects are prevalent with their use. They may include nausea, vomiting, diarrhea, insomnia, dyspepsia, anorexia, and leg cramps.

A drug that preserves acetylcholine, Galantamine (*Reminyl*), has been shown to improve the functioning of AD patients. Acetylcholine is a brain chemical vital for nerve cells to communicate with each other. Galantamine has been approved for use in Sweden and is being considered for approval in the U.S. Anti-inflammatory drugs are believed to play a role in slowing the cognitive decline of AD. Anti-inflammatory drugs such as Naproxen and Dapsone (*Aviosulfon*) are currently undergoing clinical trials to test their effect on AD patients. Memantime (Namenda) may improve memory, awareness and the ability to perform daily functions by blocking the action of a protein glutamate.

New research and on going studies that have yielded promising results include Dimebon, a Russian antihistamine, Valproic acid an epilepsy drug, nicotinamide, a form of B-3, *Remember*, a drug that dissolves tau tangles, and PBT2 that also reduces brain plaques. All not FDA approved but they have shown promise in preliminary studies.

Naturopathic therapy appears not only to address preventing AD, but also can treat it as effectively as any currently available drugs. A diet that emphasizes fruits and vegetables (antioxidants) and fish, a daily multi-vitamin/mineral, with additional supplements B-complex, C, E, PS, DHA and herbs such as ginkgo, ginseng, sage, Echinacea, and garlic, are believed to prevent, delay and treat AD as well as today's drug treatment. By supplying the body what it may be lacking in nutrients, or what is destroyed by toxins, through supplements, the individual can develop proper nervous system functioning that may slow or even prevent AD.

Side effects from naturopathic treatment usually only occurs when more than recommended amounts of supplements are taken, or when they are used in conjunction with prescription medications that may counteract or amplify the effects of the medications. Activity, both physical and mental is imperative to delay the effects of AD.

Holistic Mental Health for
Alzheimer's Disease
Specific Recommendations:

Research supports the contention that a natural diet, with additional supplements of specific vitamins, minerals and herbs can slow and possibly prevent the onset of Alzheimer's disease as well as any prescription medications currently available, without the harmful side effects. This would consist of:

- A diet of fresh vegetables, fruits, whole grains, with limited saturated fats, sugars and processed foods. Protein from cold water fish, 3 to 4 times per week (omega-3 EFA's) and lean meats like turkey or chicken breasts.

- Additional daily supplements of: multi-vitamin/mineral, B-complex (120-150 mg, per day), vitamin C (1,500 to 2,000 mg, per day), vitamin E (400 to 800 IUs, per day), Calcium (1,000 to 1,500 mg, per day), magnesium (300 to 500 mg, per day), zinc (15 to 30 mg, per day), ginkgo (120 to 240 mg, per day), Asian ginseng (150 to 250 mg, per day), DHA when not eating fish (300 mg, per day).

- Avoid consumption of alcohol (brain poison), caffeine (stimulate), nicotine (reduces oxygen supply to brain) and exposure to toxic metals like aluminum (cookware, antacids, deodorants) lead, mercury, copper, and iron.

- Exercise, physically and mentally, is often considered a "fountain of youth" as it increases the overall health of all body systems and helps the body get rid of toxins.

Treatment for medical conditions should always be conducted by your healthcare professional. According to the FDA only physicians are allowed to prescribe medications, and the suggestions in this book are for dietary changes and/or supplements only.

CHAPTER III:
ANXIETY DISORDER and STRESS:

In this age of technology stress almost appears commonplace. A generation ago valium prescriptions were the norm. Today people take xanex, and give their hyperactive children that can't sleep trazodone. Anti-anxiety medications and programs (like stress reduction) are a big business in the U.S. $42 billion is spent annually in the U.S. alone. An estimated 28.8 % of Americans will experience some kind of anxiety disorder in their lifetime, and 12.7 million women suffer from phobias, the most common form of anxiety disorder annually [1].

Anxiety disorders are the most common psychiatric illnesses in children. Childhood anxiety disorders also foreshadow psychiatric illness later in life. These disorders predict an increase by a factor of 2 to 5 times of the risk of later anxiety disorders, major depression, suicide attempts and hospitalization for psychiatric illness. Anxiety disorders with their underlying cognitive distortions (like depression), disrupt psychological development [2].

The failure to diagnose and treat anxiety disorders during adolescents can lead to social dysfunction. Adolescents are more likely to develop alcohol dependence, substance abuse, and cigarette smoking in efforts to self-medicate when they have an anxiety disorder. The lifetime risk of major depression is as high as 70 percent for patients with social phobia or generalized anxiety disorder. When combined with depression the likelihood of a suicide attempt increases by a factor of 2 to 6. Anxiety disorders are associated with increased risk of failure in school, low paying jobs, and financial dependence in the form of welfare or government subsides. Correspondingly, these disorders lead to a substantially reduced quality of life and high rates of use of mental health and medical services[3].

Lifetime prevalence rates for Panic Disorder, a type of Anxiety Disorder is estimated at 3.5 percent of the population. In medical settings the rate jumps from 10 to 30 percent of individuals seeking treatment, and up to 60 percent of those in cardiology clinics.

Anxiety Disorders most typically start during late adolescence and the mid 30's. However, in children the most commonly endorsed anxiety symptoms were over concern about competence, excessive need for reassurance, fear of the dark, fear of harm to an attachment figure, and somatic complaints. Girls generally endorse more symptoms than boys do, and younger children are more likely to experience separation anxiety than older children.

Panic Disorder typically begins in late adolescence to early adulthood. Some individuals may have episodic outbreaks of Anxiety Disorder symptoms with years of remission in between, others may have continuous severe symptomatology [4, 5]. Other conditions linked to prolonged anxiety and psychological stress include; angina, asthma, autoimmune diseases, cancer, cardiovascular disease, common cold, diabetes, depression, headaches, hypertension, irritable bowel syndrome, and ulcers [6].

Stress, a leading cause of Anxiety Disorders, account for up to 90 percent of visits to primary care physicians. Nearly one-fifth of every health clinic patient is suffering from an anxiety disorder or related illness. As many as 750,000 Americans attempt suicide each year, often due to unmanageable stress. On the average work day nearly one million employees are absent due to stress-related problems, costing American businesses more than $200 billion annually in absenteeism, worker's compensation claims, health insurance costs and lowered productivity. Up to 40 percent of employee turnover is stress-related. Recent studies have shown that stress also weakens our immune system, impairs our mood and performance, disturbs our sleep, contributes to sexual dysfunction, and destroys relationships [7].

Types of Anxiety Disorders:

Under "anxiety disorders" the DSM-IV-TR (2000) classifies the following disorders as anxiety related illnesses:

Panic Attack: A sudden onset of intense apprehension, fearfulness, or terror, often associated with feelings of impending doom. During these attacks symptoms of shortness of breath, palpitations, chest pain or discomfort, choking or smothering sensations, and fear of "going crazy" or losing control are present. A Panic Disorder (PD) is the presence of recurrent and unexpected Panic Attacks.

Agoraphobia: Anxiety about, or avoidance of, places or situations from which escape might be difficult (or embarrassing) or in which help may not be available in the event of having a Panic Attack or panic-like symptoms.

Specific Phobia: Are characterized by clinically significant anxiety provoked by exposure to a specific feared object or situation, often leading to avoidance behavior.

Social Phobia: Are characterized by clinically significant anxiety provoked by exposure to certain types of social performance situations, often leading to avoidance behavior.

Obsessive-Compulsive Disorder (OCD): Is characterized by obsessions (which cause marked anxiety or distress) and /or by compulsions (which serve to neutralize anxiety).

Posttraumatic Stress Disorder (PTSD): Characterized by the re-experiencing of an extremely traumatic event accompanied by symptoms similar to increased arousal and by avoidance of stimuli associated with the trauma.

Acute Stress Disorder: Characterized by symptoms similar to those of Posttraumatic Stress Disorder that occur immediately in the aftermath of an extremely traumatic event.

Generalized Anxiety Disorder (GAD): Characterized by at least 6 months of persistent and excessive anxiety and worry.

The above anxiety disorders can appear by themselves or in conjunction with other disorders (co morbidity). Panic Disorder is often co morbid with GAD and Social Phobia (15 to 30%), and OCD (10%). PTSD is co-morbid with Panic Disorder 10% of the time. Panic Disorder is also co-morbid with Major Depressive Disorder (MDD) from 10 to 65% of the time. In two-thirds of the time depression is coincident with or follows the onset of Panic Disorder. In the remaining one-third the depression precedes the onset of Panic Disorder [3].

Causes of Anxiety Disorders:

According to Freudian psychology, anxiety is a sign of intrapsychic conflict, usually between an unconscious wish and a learned prohibition. However, research during the past ten years has elucidated the neuronal circuitry and the molecular biology that underlie many of the manifestations of anxiety and the actions of anti-anxiety medications.

Fear Factor

Fear and anxiety are studied in animal models, which usually entail stress in the form of exposure to a potentially dangerous environment. This stimuli that is perceived dangerous on the basis of prior learning is processed by pathways leading from the thalamus and sensory cortex to specific limbic structures, particularly the amygdala and hippocampus, which are critical for the initiation and mediation of learned responses to fear. It has been shown that monkeys with lesions of the amygdala lose their fear of snakes. Humans with damage to the amygdala have difficulty perceiving fear on someone's face and do not learn normally to identify stimuli that signal danger. A recent functional neurologic imaging study has shown that physiologic activation of the amygdala occurs when a subject is shown fearful stimuli [9].

Specific neurons of the amygdala and hippocampus project widely to groups of cells that participate in the physiological and behavioral responses associated with fear and anxiety. These cells occur in regions of the hypothalamus and brain stem that mediate sympathetic and parasympathetic autonomic responses and are involved in arousal and priming behavioral responses. The neurotransmitters of these pathways include glutamate y-aminobutyric acid (GABA), serotonin, norepinephrine, and the neuroactive peptide corticotropin-releasing factor [10].

Stress

Biochemical responses to stress have been of interest to researchers for decades. For years scientists were focused on the role of the adrenal glands, the small organs on top of the kidneys. They produce a hormone that is activated in times of severe stress, adrenaline. Adrenaline, named after the gland that produces it (or the scientific name of epinephrine) is also called the "fight-or-flight" hormone. It was the role of adrenaline in the body's handling of stress that led scientists to study the effects of norepinephrine and its role as a neurotransmitter.

Another chemical produced by the adrenal glands, cortisol, is known to be released in times of stress. Cortisol is sometimes called the "stress hormone" and elevated levels have been found in the blood of severely depressed individuals. In autopsies performed on patients who have died from suicide have also shown enlarged adrenal glands. As scientists investigated the mechanisms that cause the release of stress hormones they discovered that there is a cascade of the release of hormones beginning in the brain. At the top of the cascade is a substance produced in the brain called corticotropin-releasing factor (CRF). Elevated CRF levels can be measured in the brains of rats subjected to stress [11].

By applying the kindling model of behavior to the biochemistry of the brain scientists begin to explain the how anxiety and stress occurs. The kindling model explains how in some instances individuals become sensitive to less stimuli. This model works opposite to most biological processes that use a negative feedback loop, in which a system needs ever-increasing stimulus to elicit a response.

For example, an addict of street drugs may require progressively larger fixes to obtain the same "high". The kindling model of stress explains how stimuli can build to where it takes less stimuli to elicit a larger response. Combining the kindling model with changes in brain chemistry during stress or anxiety (elevated levels of CRF) it is believed that psychosocial stressors like pain, isolation, confinement and lack of control can lead to structural changes in the brain and can kindle progressively more autonomous acute symptoms [12].

Environmental Causes

Dr. Carl Pfeiffer, director of the Brain Bio Center in New Jersey has treated thousands of patients since the 1960's through the connection between mental illness and biochemistry. His research showed a relationship between low levels of blood histamine and mental disorders such as schizophrenia. Histamine is a brain chemical responsible for a number of body functions such as reaction to pain, and allergies and the production of body secretions like mucus and saliva. Low blood histamine levels are also linked to high levels of copper, thus both are believed to be linked to behavioral abnormalities.

High copper levels may be caused by environmental factors such as copper water pipes or copper cookware. The high levels of copper cause behavioral abnormalities characterized by anxiety, extreme fears, paranoia and hallucinations. High levels of copper also deplete vitamins C and B_3. Dr. Pfeiffer's clinic has successfully treated such behavioral disorders with manganese and zinc which counteracts copper in the blood stream and increased vitamins C and B_3 which is depleted by high copper levels [13].

Biochemical Causes

Biochemical causes of panic attacks are believed to be linked to lactic acid metabolism. Lactic acid is produced when the body burns glucose, or blood sugar without oxygen. This is done usually during vigorous exercise when not enough oxygen is taken in. Lactic acid is changed into lactate and transported to the liver, where it is converted to harmless pyruvic acid.

People who suffer from panic attacks, however, are unable to convert lactate into pyruvic acid, and so have elevated blood levels of lactate. Alcohol and sugar consumption also can increase the production of lactate in the body. Other nutritional factors of anxiety and stress include excessive coffee consumption, or a deficiency of alphalinolenic acid, and essential omega-3 fatty acid [14].

Genetic Causes

There is evidence to suggest that anxiety disorders have genetic factors. Research indicates that mothers with elevated levels of anxiety, panic disorder and depression had infants with markedly anxious temperaments and high levels of anxiety when placed in new settings. These responses persisted into adolescents and early adulthood.

Studies of families and twins indicate the important influence of heritable risk factors. Some of the genes that confer an increased risk of anxiety disorders may be shared with those that increase the risk of a Major Depressive Disorder (MDD), thus explaining the high rate of co morbidity of these disorders [15].

Allopathic Treatment for Anxiety Disorders:

Anxiety is as old as mankind, and attempts to cure this subjective uneasiness by ingesting something is just as old. The earliest self-medicating strategy involved alcohol. Today in the 21st century, alcohol is still the most commonly self-prescribed treatment for anxiety. Many compounds historically used to treat anxiety were neither safe nor effective.

Early Treatment

Bromo-seltzers were proclaimed a long-term treatment in the 1900's but bromide dependency became a significant problem, and these products were withdrawn from the market. Subsequently, barbiturates were developed as a potentially safe class of drugs. However, they too were found to develop adverse effects such as seizures, the potential for addiction, dependence and withdrawal. Other compounds developed at the time such as opioids and tincture of belladonna, also had significant problems of abuse and dependence [16].

A major advance following barbiturates was the development of meprobamate in the mid 1950's. this drug was also found to be highly addictive. The first benzodiazepine, chlordiazepoxide (Librium), appeared on the scene in the 1960's. introduced with the promise of efficacy and safety, withdrawal symptoms were observed similar to that of meprobamate and barbiturates.

In 1986 buspirone (BuSpar), a structurally unique nonbenzodiazepine anti-anxiety drug, was introduced. This drug reportedly does not have the tolerance and dependency and the complications of previously prescribed anti-anxiety medications [17].

Current Psychopharmacology

Today psychopharmacology of anxiety disorders includes treatment with anti-anxiety agents and hypnotics, known collectively as sedative-hypnotics. Anti-anxiety medications are non-sedating and primarily used to treat daytime tension, whereas, hypnotics relieve insomnia. Anti-anxiety medications include benzodiazepines, buspirone, clomipramine, clonidine, hydroxyzine, meprobamate, propranolol, and trazodone [18].

Benzodiazepines

Of the various neurochemical agents used to treat symptoms of anxiety, benzodiazepines are the most broadly effective. Some common benzodiazepines include Alprazolam *(Xanax)*, Clonazepam *(Klonopin)*, Lorazepam *(Ativan)*, and Diazepam *(Valium)*. The brain has specific binding sites for benzodiazepines, and the actions of these agents are mediated at GABA receptors, where they potentiate the inhibitory effects of GABA.

In animal studies it is found that the infusion of benzodiazepines directly into the amygdala blocks fear conditioning and the physiological response to perceived danger. However, because GABA receptors are widely distributed in the brain, benzodiazepines modify the effects of GABA in many brain circuits and therefore have diverse effects, such as sedative or hypnotic effects, anticonvulsant actions, and muscle-relaxant effects, they may also cause ataxia and amnesia. Other side effects include physiological and psychological dependence [19, 20].

Clonidine

Clonidine is used for panic attacks but has many side effects. Side effects reported with use include cardiac disorders, moderate to severe hypertension, and metabolic or renal disease. Propranolol, a β-blocker, is most useful against the physical signs of "flight or fight" response such as heart palpitations, tachycardia, GI upset, tremors and sweating. Unlike benzodiazepines, propranolol does not dim consciousness, cause drowsiness or produce drug dependency. However, propranolol may cause fatigue and depression, liver and kidney impairment, and should not be used by diabetics as it complicates carbohydrate and fat metabolism. Buspirone hydrochloride (Buspar) is used for Generalized Anxiety Disorder, social phobias, OCD, and PTSD, and does not cause drug dependence like benzodiazepines, and has fewer side effects. Like many antidepressants it takes 4 to 6 weeks to be effective [21, 22].

Antihistamines

Antihistamines are prescribed for anxiety due their sedating effects. Examples of antihistamines include hydroxyzine hydrochloride (Atarax) used for common anxiety and tension. Antihistamines work by decreasing the effects of histamine, a chemical in the body that narrows air passages in the lungs and contributes to inflammation. Antihistamines also relieve itching and swelling, and dry up secretions from the nose, eyes, and throat. They are not usually recommended for long-term use and side effects could include drowsiness, dry mouth, twitches, tremors, and convulsions [23, 24].

Antidepressants

Many antidepressants are also prescribed for anxiety disorders. Tricyclic antidepressants (TCAs), like clomipramine (*Anafranil*), and selective serotonin reuptake inhibitors (SSRIs), such as paroxetine (*Paxil*), fluoxetine (*Prozac*), fluvoxamine (*Luvox*), sertraline (*Zoloft*), and venlafaxine (*Effexor*), have been used to treat GAD, panic disorder, phobic disorders, obsessive-compulsive disorder, and post-traumatic stress disorder. However, antidepressants typically take 2 to 4 weeks for a response and side effects range from mild (dry mouth, nausea, headaches) to severe (seizures, liver damage, heart rate fluctuations, hypertension, strokes, death). Venlafaxine can be fatal if taken with MAOIs [25, 26, 27].

Newer antidepressants have been found to be effective in treating anxiety. Alprazolam (*Xanax*) and adinazolam are antidepressants that have been found to have a sedating effect and is useful in agitation and panic disorders. Side effects of Alprazolam and adinazolam may be that they are possibly addictive, and could have withdrawal seizures [28, 29].

In a recent study, fluvoxamine (*Luvox*), a selective serotonin reuptake inhibitor was evaluated for effectiveness in treating anxiety disorders. In the study, 128 children ages 6 to 17 years-old who had diagnosis of social phobia, separation anxiety disorder or generalized anxiety disorder, were given either 300 mg of fluvoxamine or a placebo for 8 weeks. Both groups received supportive psychotherapy also. It was found that the children who received the fluvoxamine had a substantial reduction in anxiety symptoms, whereas the children in the placebo group did not. Eight percent of the children in the fluvoxmine group dropped out due to adverse side effects, compared to 2 percent of the placebo group [30].

Quetiapine fumarate (Seroquel), and antipsychotic drug that is usually prescribed to treat schizophrenia and bipolar disorder may also ease GAD. A study with 854 patients with Generalized Anxiety Disorder showed improvement of reducing their anxiety when taking Seroquel XR. Most common side effects in that study were dry mouth, insomnia, sedation, dizziness, nausea and headache [31].

Behavior Therapy

The medical community appears divided over the recommended course of treatment for anxiety disorders. A number of well designed studies support the use of non-pharmacological treatments for anxiety disorders. Psychological interventions such as relaxation training, anxiety management and cognitive behavior therapy, are effective and may reduce symptoms for at least one year.

Cognitive behavior therapy involves such strategies as desensitization and positive mental imaging to reduce a patient's anxiety about feared situations. Because patients with anxiety disorders who also had depression were typically excluded from studies of psychological intervention, the broad effectiveness of these treatments in clinical practice remains uncertain. Such coexisting disorders are believed to even reduce the efficacy of treatment. No direct comparisons have been made between selective serotonin reuptake inhibitors and psychological treatments in children with anxiety disorders. Therefore, doctors appear uncertain which approach is superior. However, given that the rates of response to either treatment appear to be roughly similar, cognitive behavior therapy may be preferred to pharmacotherapy as an initial treatment because of the low risk of side effects [32].

Table 3-1
Summary of Allopathic Treatment for Anxiety Disorders:

Drug: (Brand name)	Acting mechanism:	Possible side effects:
Benzodiazepines: **Alprazolam** *(Xanax),* **Ativan** *(Lorazepam),* **Clonazepam** *(Klonopin),* **Clorazepate dipotassium** *(Tranxene),* **Diazepam** *(Valium),* **Oxazepam**	Inhibits GABA receptors in the brain.	Sedative and hypnotic effects, may cause ataxia and amnesia, physiological and psychological dependence. Possible liver damage, headache, nausea, rash, fluid retention, tremors.
Propranolol *(Apo-propranolol, Detensol, inderal, Novopranol)*	Relaxes physiological processes such as sympathetic nervous system, reduces heart rate, blood pressure, muscle cells of small arteries.	Dry mouth, weak pulse, vomiting, muscle cramps, mood changes, nausea, dizziness, depression, sexual dysfunction, constipation, diarrhea, insomnia, headache, appetite loss, seizures, irregular heartbeat, anxiety.
Buspirone hydrochloride *(Buspar)*	May regulate neurotransmitters. Not as sedating or addictive as Benzodiazepines.	Headache, nausea, dizziness, dry mouth, depression, agitation.
Antihistamines: **Diphenhydramine** *(Benadryl),* **Hydroxyzine** *(Atarax)*	Sedating action on the nervous system reduces anxiety.	Drowsiness, dizziness, dry mouth, loss of appetite, nightmares, agitation, irritability, fatigue, weakness, fainting, seizures.

Tricyclic anti-depressants: Amitriptyline hydrochloride (Triavil) Clomipramine (Anafranil). Doxepin hydrochloride (Sinequan)	Blocks neurotransmitter (serotonin) reuptake.	Tremor, headache, dry mouth, constipation or diarrhea, nausea, anxiety, indigestion, fatigue, insomnia, dizziness, decreased sex drive, hallucinations.
SSRIs: Escitalopram oxalate (Lexapro), Fluoxetine (Prozac), Fluvoxamine (Luvox), Paroxetine (Paxil), Sertraline (Zoloft), Venlafaxine (Effexor)	Inhibits the reuptake of serotonin in the brain.	Drowsiness, nausea, constipation or diarrhea, headache, anxiety, sexual dysfunction, insomnia, dry mouth, confusion, apathy, heartbeat irregularity, muscle or joint pain, hair loss.
Atypical Antidepressants: Bupropion (Wellbutrin), Nefazodone (Serzone), Trazodone (Desyrel)	Increases neurotransmitter activity.	Blurred vision, increased heart rate and blood pressure, insomnia, dizziness, nausea, headache, dry mouth, decreased sexual drive, seizures.

Naturopathic Treatment for Anxiety Disorders:

Naturopathic treatment or what is termed alternative medicine or complementary medicine, is now making its way into the western medical practice mainstream. Medical schools now teach alternative medicine, hospitals and health maintenance organizations offer it and laws in some states require health plans to cover it. Even major pharmaceutical companies are starting to get involved in the herbal treatment revolution. Of all the forms of alternative treatments, the most common is herbal medicine [33].

Dr. Isaacs questions the 1999 Surgeon General's report on mental health, which states that "approximately one in five children and adolescents experiences the signs and symptoms of a DSM-IV disorder during the course of a year," and emphasizes that we have increasingly relabeled troublesome behavior and emotional distress in children as mental illness, which can and should be treated with drugs. She states that the large number of researchers making these claims cannot offer any evidence that psychopharmacologic treatments do not affect the developing brains of young children, over the short or long term. And, most researchers attribute the difficulties of childhood to defective genes or neurological systems of the children, rather than environmental causes of psychological disorders like stress on families, poor living conditions or a poor school environment. She believes that although a small number of severely disturbed children may need drug treatment, that we are pacifying millions of our children to avoid dealing with larger social issues [34].

Ginseng

Studies on herbs are becoming more prevalent in support of their treatment for mental disorders. **Ginseng**, has been used for centuries to boost energy, sharpen the mind, reduce stress, reverse impotence, and extend life. There are several different species of ginseng used medicinally in the genus *Panax,* but the two most popular are **Asian ginseng**, *Panax ginseng,* and **American ginseng**, *Panax quinquefolius.*

Asian ginseng is also called Oriental, Chinese or Korean ginseng and is considered a warm, stimulating "yang" tonic. It should be avoided by people who are nervous or anxious unless they are using it to boost their energy. American ginseng is a cooling, sedating "yin" tonic that helps bring balance and harmony to the body. It used to reduce stress and anxiety, and calm the body. Ginseng's medicinal properties are concentrated its thick, fleshy root that resembles a white or yellow carrot [35].

Although herbalists have used ginseng for thousands of years it was not "clinically" tested until the 1960's. At that time a study from the Soviet Union showed how mice treated with ginseng had increased endurance and energy. A search then ensued to isolate and analyze the active ingredients in ginseng. What were discovered were compounds known as terpenoidal glycosides, which are sugar molecules attached to plant hormones. Ginseng glycosides form in the leaves, flowers and outer coating of the root, and then they are stored in the root. Up to 6 percent of the dried root can contain glycosides. A Japanese researcher coined the phrase ginsenoside to describe these glycosides in 1961. More than 20 different ginsenosides have been identified in various species of ginseng. Ginsenosides in ginseng is believed to reduce stress by increasing the blood flow to the brain, improving concentration and mental performance [36].

A number of studies have supported ginseng's effectiveness as a mood enhancing treatment. Researchers at the University of Goteberg, Sweden gave 480 older individuals ginseng or a placebo. The group on ginseng was reported to be significantly more relaxed, had better moods, had more energy and were more alert than the placebo group. A number of animal studies support ginseng's use in treating stress. Studies in labs in England, Korea, Russia, and the U.S. have shown that ginseng helps mice tolerate stressful situations. After taking ginseng the mice were better able to 'absorb stress" with out experiencing distress or abnormal behavior. Animals that took ginseng not only coped better with stressful situations but their body activity settled back to normal more quickly [37].

For ginseng to be effective it should contain between 3 to 6 percent ginsenosides by weight. Ginseng comes in pill form, teas, powders, tinctures, or raw roots. Recommended daily doses of ginseng is one gram per day. Most side effects of ginseng do not occur with recommended does. However when excessive amounts are taken side effects may include diarrhea, diminished libido, earaches, headaches, high blood pressure, insomnia, rashes, nosebleeds, and vomiting [38].

Individuals on MAOIs for depression such as phenelzine (Nardil) should not take Asian ginseng, *Panax ginseng,* as reports of hypomania have occurred when combining the two. Excessive vaginal bleeding has been reported when Asian ginseng is taken with ticlopidine *(Ticlid),* a platelet inhibiting drug used to prevent stroke. Similar findings have been reported with Asian ginseng and warfarin *(Coumadin)* an anticoagulant used to treat blood clots [39].

Kava kava

Another herbaceous root that has been used to relieve anxiety and stress for hundreds of years is **Kava kava,** *Piper methysticum.* The herb is native to the Polynesia and Melanesia islands of the South Pacific where the root is brewed into a relaxing tea and used in island ceremonies. Kava has been used in the West for more than 200 years, since James Cook, the eighteenth-century British explorer, brought the plant back to Europe.

Researchers first began looking into the relaxant properties of kava in the 1950's and recent clinical studies have supported its use in treating anxiety and stress. Kava appears to work by modifying rather than blocking brain chemicals that affect emotions. This is unlike prescription anti-anxiety drugs that produce a calming effect by blocking these neurochemicals. However, when these neurochemicals are blocked by medications other senses are dulled especially mental alertness. Kava elevates mood and increases mental alertness.

The active ingredients in kava responsible for its calming effect are called kavalactones, and are extracted from the herb's root. Commercial preparations of kava are standardized to range in potency from 3 to 30 percent kavalactones. Taken internally kava is available as dried root, tincture (liquid), tea, and capsules. *Kavapyrone* tablets of 60 to 120 mg is recommended. Dr. David

Williams recommends 50 mg of kavalactones 3 times per day for anxiety, and 150 to 200 mg all at once an hour before bedtime for insomnia.

Teas are often combined with other calming herbs such as chamomile, lavender, or passionflower. High doses of kava have reported to have side effects of skin, nail and hair discoloration, scaly skin, swollen face and eyes, muscle weakness, and motor and vision problems. Kava use should not be combined with alcohol, conventional anti-anxiety drugs, or sleep medication [40, 41].

Lavender

Lavender, *Lavandula officinalis,* is considered an aromatic healing herb. Lavender has a long history of commercial use in soaps, bath products, perfumes, powders, sachets, and moth repellants. Therapeutic properties of lavender are used in relieving stress and anxiety, tension, insomnia, headache and nausea. Taken internally lavender is available as teas, dried flowers, powdered herb, capsules and tinctures. Externally, the essential oil of lavender is used in aromatherapy to promote relaxation, stimulate the mind clarify thinking, encourage creativity, and relieve depression [42].

Skullcap/Virginian

Skullcap/Virginian, *Scutellaria lateriflora,* has been used as a remedy for sleep disorders and as a tranquilizer. The leaves and blue flowers of the Virginian species of skullcap have long been used in many herbal sleep remedies and tranquilizing teas. Native Americans regularly used skullcap as a sedative and indigestion treatment. Some holistic practitioners believe that skullcap is particularly effective in neutralizing negative emotions, like anger, and is helpful in enhancing the meditative state.

Skullcap is available as a dried herb, tea, tincture, and capsules. Hot tea is especially effective in treating anxiety and tension. In tablet form 250 to 500 mg, 3 times a day is recommended. Side effects of skullcap could include upset stomachs, diarrhea, twitching, convulsions or drowsiness if too much is taken [43, 44].

Valerian

Valerian, *Valeriana officinalis,* is often thought of as the "valium" of the plant kingdom. It has been used for over the 1,000 years as a relaxant. Modern medical literature records the use of valerian for anxiety in the 19th century in the *New American Family Physician* (1883) listing the herb as a remedy for nervousness.

Recent research has confirmed valerian as a mild and safe tranquilizer that is particularly useful for treating anxiety, nervous tension, stress and panic attacks. Valerian is also reported as a good treatment as a sleep aid where, unlike pharmaceutical sedatives it does not interfere with dream states or rapid eye movement. Valerian is taken internally for anxiety, nervousness, and tension, stress related headache, muscle ache, and internal pains, menstrual cramps, and insomnia.

Valerian is available as a dried herb, capsules, tincture, and teas, alone or in combination with other calming herbs such as St. John's wort, passionflower or Kava kava. Recommended dosage in *Valepotriate* tablets is 50 mg, 3 times a day. Over consumption of the herb may lead to headache, restlessness, nausea, drowsiness or blurred vision. It should not be used when on prescription tranquilizers or sedatives due to additive effect [45, 46, 47].

Chamomile

Chamomile, *Matricaria chamomilla,* was reported to be first used by the ancient Egyptians and has been used for thousands of years since. Its common name is derived from the Greek word *chamai* (on the ground) and *melon* (apple) to mean "ground apple", a dual reference to how the plant grows on the ground and has an apple scent. Of the two most common varieties of chamomile German and Roman chamomile, the German variety is the most popular and thoroughly studied.

Researchers believe elements in the oil of the flowers, primarily apigenin and azulene are responsible for calming the central nervous system, relax the digestive track, speed healing and fight infection. Chamomile is also rich in calcium, magnesium, and iron. The warm tea is calming and helps induce relaxation and promote sleep. Soaking in a chamomile bath will not only calm nerves it will also relieve minor aches and pains.

Taken internally, as in teas chamomile has sedating properties, antispasmodic, pain-relieving and wound-healing properties. Chamomile is used as dried or fresh flowers, tea, tincture, and essential oil. It is often combined with other herbs for relaxation and sleep such as Kava kava, valerian and passionflower. People who have ragweed allergies may also have allergic reactions to chamomile other adverse side effects have not been reported [48, 49].

Lemon balm

Lemon balm, *Melissa officinalis,* is a close relative to chamomile. It is the mildest of the sedating herbs and is often prescribed for children. It is especially effective in relaxing the body and calming the emotions prior to sleep. Lemon balm is a lemon scented member of the mint the family and was favored daily toddy in 16th and 17th century England.

Several modern studies have originated from Germany for its medicinal effects. Therapeutically lemon balm has antispasmodic action, is mildly sedating, and relieves indigestion. Lemon balm's sedating action seems to specifically to target brain activity, and is frequently prescribed for insomnia, or other sleep problems in which there is anxiety, stress, depression, or hyperactivity.

In Germany, it is the main ingredient of a popular medicine, *Melissengeist,* which is prescribed for those symptoms. Taken internally for restlessness, insomnia, anxiety, headaches, depression, and heart palpitations, lemon balm is available as a dried herb, tincture, tea, capsules and oil. Teas are often combined with chamomile, valerian or passionflower for calming sleep aids. Lemon balm has no reported side effects, however, it should not be used by people with thyroid-related conditions [50, 51].

Passionflower

Passionflower, *Passiflora incarnata,* was named by Spanish explorers who saw in its flowers' ornate design elements of the "passion" or suffering, of Jesus. Native Americans in the southeastern United States, particularly the Cherokee, used the pleasant tasting herb in healing. It was introduced to Europe in the late 1800's for its calming effect on the central nervous system. The flower, vine and leaves of this herb contain alkaloids and flavonoids that, in laboratory studies, have demonstrated sedating effects.

Herbalist recommend passionflower as a sedative, digestive aid or pain reliever. Passionflower also reduces high blood pressure. It is most used for chronic stress relief, anxiety and insomnia. Because it dilates blood vessels it is being tested as a heart disease preventive. Passionflower used as dried or fresh leaves, capsules, tea or tincture. For anxiety 1 dropper of tincture in warm water four times a day is recommended. Passionflower should not be used with other prescription sedatives as over medication can occur, and pregnant women should not use it as it may stimulate uterine muscles. Mild side effects of upset stomach, nausea, vomiting, diarrhea, and sleepiness may occur with overuse [52, 53, 54].

Nutritional Supplementation

Nutritional intervention may be very effective in relieving anxiety. If anxiety is due to lactate metabolism difficulties, calcium and magnesium (800 to 1,200 mg, per day) will help lower lactate production. B-complex supplements also decrease lactate. Alcohol and sugar consumption should be reduced to help lower lactate production as well. Alpha-linolenic acid (ALA), an essential omega-3 fatty acid supplementation has been shown to be effective in treating anxiety. In a study of patients with agoraphobia (fear of going outdoors) 3 out of 4 people improved after two months when taking 2 to 3 teaspoons of flaxseed oil (high in ALA) per day.

Excess caffeine consumption can increase stress levels all day. Research has shown significant decrease in stress symptoms when coffee consumption is eliminated for a week. Sugar consumption depletes nutrients from the body and eventually will burn out the adrenals. Symptoms of adrenal exhaustion are anxiety, depression, chronic fatigue, low stress tolerance and irritability.

Reducing sugar and increasing the intake of vitamins A, C, B-complex, E, and calcium and selenium aids in stress reduction. Potassium is needed for proper adrenal gland function and is found in high amounts in foods like potatoes, avocados, bananas, tomatoes and fish. Pantothenic acid is also important for the adrenal gland, and is found in whole grains, legumes, cauliflower, broccoli, salmon, liver, sweet potatoes and tomatoes.

Magnesium is needed in order for calcium to function in the nerves and is found in green foods that are rich in chlorophyll People who eat diets high in carbohydrates of whole, natural foods such as vegetables, grains and fruits invariably are calm, rarely depressed and able to sleep soundly [55, 56, 57, 58, 59, 60, 61].

A study from the University of California found that lack of a brain protein can lead to insomnia and stress. Neuropeptide S, is a protein produced in parts of the brain that regulate arousal and anxiety. When researchers gave mice injections of neuropeptide S they exhibited far less stress or sleep disturbances [62].

Alternative Therapies:

Yoga

Alternative therapies such as yoga have been shown to treat anxiety and stress. Studies have indicated that anxiety disorders such as obsessive-compulsive disorder (OCD) have been reduced to the point of not requiring medication after yoga therapy for three to twelve months [63]. It is believed that yoga dates back as far as 20,000 BC. Contemporary yoga was reorganized as a philosophy 500 years ago.

Today there are two main types of yoga, **Raja Yoga,** and **Hatha Yoga**. Raja Yoga attempts to achieve self-realization through spiritual discipline, a strict practice of meditation, diet and moderation living. Hatha Yoga attains self-realization through perfection of the body by physical exercise, breathing exercises, stretching and relaxation techniques. Despite the many types of yoga the benefits of sustained practice include relief from daily pressures, relaxation, feeling grounded and connected to the body, improved muscle and skin tone, healthy internal organs, weight loss, improved circulation, flexibility relief from stiffness and insomnia and increased stamina [64]. Studies have also revealed anxiety reducing results with **Transcendental Meditation**, a type of meditation used in Ayurvedic medicine [65].

Hypnotherapy

Hypnotherapy has been shown to be highly effective in treating anxiety, stress and specific phobias. Hypnotherapy practices date back thousands of years, and employs the power of suggestion to heal the body or mind. Hypnotherapy has gained increasing acceptance in the medical community in the past 100 years due to the efforts of Clark Hull who promoted controlled hypnosis research, and Milton Erickson who founded the American Society of Clinical Hypnosis (ASCH) in 1957. The ASCH is a society of professionals in the medical, psychological and dental professions dedicated to informing the public about the therapeutic effects of hypnosis.

When treating anxiety, stress and phobias the hypnotherapist places the patient in a trance state by relaxing the body and then they attempt to re-program the subconscious. By suggesting relaxing techniques or using guided meditation the hypnotherapist relaxes the patient and then implants healing suggestions. Hypnotherapy has been shown to be a proven technique as an adjunct or primary therapy for a wide range of medical and psychological disorders [66, 67].

Meditation

Deep meditation produces a state called blanking out. It can be achieved by meditation, as in yoga, **Zen Meditation** or in deep prayer. This blanking out or a turning off point of consciousness is believed to be based on how our central nervous system functions. By restricting attention to one unchanging source of stimulation a 'turning off' of consciousness of the external world follows.

By whatever means blanking out occurs it has significant effects on reducing stress and anxiety. Levels of stress-related biochemicals such as adrenaline and cortisol are dramatically decreased, blood pressure and heart rate also decrease. Blanking out allows brainwaves to become synchronized between the brain's two hemispheres producing gains in certain types of mental functioning such as memory and concentration, and deep relaxation is achieved [68].

A device that produces a blanking out condition was developed by neurophysiologist, Dr. John Lilly, called the floatation tank. A floatation tank is an enclosed container about the size of a small closet turned on its side. It contains a shallow pool of water about ten inches deep that is saturated with dissolved Epsom salts creating a dense solution that allows anyone laying in it to float like a cork. When the door of the tank is closed it is totally dark creating an immediate visual blanking out. The individual's ear are also plugged creating an absence of external sounds. The floatation in body temperature water gives the feeling of weightlessness and makes the effect of total sensory deprivation complete.

Significant research has been conducted on the positive relaxing effects the floatation tank produces. Studies from the Medical College of Ohio, Lawrence College, St. Elizabeth's Hospital in Appleton, Wisconsin, and the University of British Columbia demonstrate that floating has a dramatic stress-reduction effect. Among the findings are that periodic floats reduce heart rate, oxygen consumption, and the levels of stress-related biochemicals in the blood stream, including cortisol, ACTH, lactate, and adrenaline.

The studies show that it not only reduces these biochemical levels during floating, but also keeps the levels low for days and in some cases weeks after the float session. Floating is believed to lower the stress-related biochemicals by causing the body to vasodilate, lowering blood pressure and increasing the flow of blood and oxygen to the brain. Floating is also believed to increase the body's tolerance for stress. Due to the relaxing effect of the float chamber has for an extended period of time after the float session it is believed to lower the set point of the endocrine homeostatic mechanism. This allows the individual to experience a lower adrenal activation state and obtain a greater degree of relaxation [69].

In clinical studies by Jon Kabot-Zinn, Ph.D founder and director of the Stress Reduction Clinic at the University of Massachusetts Medical Center it was observed that patients that underwent training in meditation had significant reductions in depression and anxiety. Dr. Kabot-Zinn's 8 week program at the clinic teaches patients techniques of mindfulness meditation, derived from the Buddhist tradition, that is guided moment to moment awareness. Patients referred to the clinic often with chronic headaches, back pain, heart disease, cancer or AIDS to learn how to relax and cope better with the stress in their lives. However, they often leave with less severe physical symptoms, and with greater self-confidence, optimism, and assertiveness. They become less anxious, less angry and less depressed over their lives [70].

Aromatherapy

Aromatherapy is using the essential oil of plants to promote healing or well being. Aromatherapy dates back a thousand years to the Arabic countries who are credited with discovering the process of distillation of oils. Essential oils are used in bath oils and soaps, perfumes and massage oils.

Several **essential oils** are used to treat anxiety. The essential oils of Clary Sage, Lavender, Jasmine, Melissa (Lemon Balm), Neroli, Marjoram, Rose, and Ylang-Ylang are recommended for stress relief baths or as massage oils [71, 72]. Research at the *University of Miami School of Medicine* used electroencephalogram (EEG) measurements to confirm aromatherapy's direct effects on the brain. They found that aromatherapy with lavender causes the brain to produce more beta waves, increased relaxation, lifting depression, and even enabling participants to solve math problems more accurately [73].

Recent clinical studies have also shown that **therapeutic massage** can alleviate stress. Combining massage with aromatherapy by using essential oils such as encourages relaxation and improves mental outlook [74].

Table 3-2
Summary of Naturopathic Treatment for Anxiety Disorders [23, 26, 42] :

Common Name/

(scientific name):

	Acting mechanism:	*Possible side effects/ Interactions:*
American Ginseng (*Panax quinquefolis*)	Active compounds of ginsenosides increases blood flow in the brain.	Toxicity side effects may include diarrhea, diminished libido, earaches, headaches, high blood pressure, insomnia, rashes, nosebleeds, vomiting. No drug interactions.
Kava kava (*Piper methysticum*)	Active compounds of kavalactones modify neurotransmitters, increases mental alertness and elevates mood.	Toxicity can cause skin, nail and hair discoloration, scaly skin, swollen eyes and face, muscle weakness, motor and vision problems. Negative interactions with alcohol, anti-anxiety and sleep medications (benzodiazepines).
Lavender (*Lavandula officinalis*)	Aromatic properties relieves stress, anxiety, insomnia, headache, nausea.	None.
Skullcap/virginian (*Scutellaria later flora*)	Nervous system sedative.	Toxicity could cause upset stomach, diarrhea, tics, convulsions, drowsiness. No drug interactions.

Valerian *(Valeriana officinalis)*	Central nervous system relaxant.	Toxicity may cause headache, restlessness, nausea, drowsiness, or blurred vision. Complimentary effects with prescription anti-anxiety medications.
Chamomile *(Matricaria chamomilla)*	Active ingredients of apigenin and azulene are responsible for calming the central nervous system.	Individuals with ragweed allergies may also have allergic reactions (hay fever, runny nose, congestion).
Lemon balm *(Melissa officinalis)*	Sedating action targets brain activity, frequently prescribed for insomnia, anxiety, depression, or hyperactivity.	Interactions with Thyroid medications.
Passionflower *(Passiflora incarnata)*	Alkaloids and flavonoids have sedating effects on the central nervous system.	Toxicity effects of upset stomach, nausea, vomiting, diarrhea, and sleepiness, pregnant woman should avoid. No drug interactions.
Alpha-linolenic acid *(ALA)*	Required for proper nervous system functioning.	None.

CONCLUSIONS:

Anxiety disorders are the most common mental disorders of children, increase the risk of later psychiatric disorders such as depression, and often lead adolescents and adults to self-medicate. Anxiety related illnesses may take the form of Panic Attacks, Agoraphobia, Specific Phobias, Social Phobias, Obsessive-Compulsive Disorder, Posttraumatic Stress Disorder, Acute Stress Disorder, or Generalized Anxiety Disorder. Anxiety disorders can appear individually or co morbid with other anxiety disorders or Major Depressive Disorder.

Causes of anxiety are believed to be a combination of environmental and biological factors. Environmental factors are connected with reaction to stressful stimuli such as pain, isolation, confinement or lack of control.

Continued stressful stimuli have a building or kindling effect that leads to an increased response to less stressful stimuli. These stressors can lead to biochemical changes in the brain from increased levels of adrenaline, cortisol, and CRF, that effect the proper functioning of neurotransmitter like serotonin, norepinephrine, and GABA. Improper lactic acid metabolism may lead to elevated levels of lactate in the blood causing Panic Attacks. A poor diet high in sugar, alcohol and coffee, and low in essential omega-3 fatty acids can increase this condition. Environmental toxins such as copper can lower blood histamine levels and deplete vitamins B3 and C, causing anxiety. Genetics also play a role in anxiety. Studies have show that parents that have elevated levels of anxiety, Panic Disorder or depression have children with higher anxiety levels then those that do not. Specific genes that are linked to MDD have also been connected to anxiety disorders.

Allopathic treatment of anxiety involves prescription anti-anxiety medications. Anti-anxiety medications such as benzodiazepines act on GABA receptors in the brain. By modifying the effects of GABA sedative, hypnotic, anticonvulsant and muscle relaxant effects occur. However, side effects of ataxia, amnesia and physiological and psychological dependence can occur. Another anti-anxiety, Clonidine, is used for treatment of panic attacks, but can cause side effects of cardiac disorders, hypertension, metabolic or renal disease. Propranolol is effective for the physical signs of anxiety such as heart palpitations, tachycardia, GI upset, tremors and sweating. Unlike benzodiazepines, Propranolol does not produce drowsiness or drug dependence, but side effects may include fatigue, depression, liver and kidney impairment. Buspirone hydrochloride (*Buspar*) is used for GAD, social phobias, OCD, and PTSD, and does not cause drug dependence like benzodiazepines, and has fewer side effects, but like many antidepressants it takes 4 to 6 weeks to be effective.

Antihistamines also have sedating effects and hydroxyzine hydrochloride is used for common anxiety and tension. Antihistamines work by decreasing the effects of histamine, a chemical in the body that narrows air passages in the lungs and contributes to inflammation. They are not usually recommended for long-term use and side effects could include drowsiness, dry mouth, twitches, tremors, and convulsions.

Antidepressants are prescribed for anxiety disorders such as TCAs, and SSRIs, and have been used to treat GAD, panic disorder, phobic disorders, obsessive-compulsive disorder, and post-traumatic stress disorder. However, antidepressants typically take 2 to 4 weeks for a response and side effects range from mild (dry mouth, nausea, headaches) to severe (seizures, liver damage, heart rate fluctuations, hypertension, stokes, death).

Newer antidepressants have been found to be effective in treating anxiety.

Alprazolam and adinazolam are antidepressants that have been found to have a sedating effect and are useful in agitation and panic disorders. Side effects of Alprazolam and adinazolam could include addiction, and withdrawal seizures. Venlafaxine hydrochloride, can be fatal if taken with MAOIs.

Non-medication treatment for anxiety usually involves psychological treatment. Psychological interventions include relaxation training, anxiety management and cognitive behavior therapy. Cognitive behavior therapy uses strategies such as desensitization and positive mental imaging to reduce a patient's anxiety about feared situations. Because patients with anxiety disorders who also had depression were typically excluded from studies of psychological intervention, the broad effectiveness of these treatments in clinical practice remains uncertain. Such coexisting disorders are believed to even reduce the efficacy of treatment. No direct comparisons have been made between SSRIs and psychological treatments in children with anxiety disorders. Therefore, doctors appear uncertain which approach is superior. However, given that the rates of response to either treatment appear to be roughly similar, cognitive behavior therapy may be preferred to pharmacotherapy as an initial treatment because of the low risk of side effects.

Naturopathic treatment for anxiety disorders uses what Western medicine calls alternative medicine or complementary medicine. It involves treatment with herbal medicine, nutritional intervention, therapeutic exercise like yoga or meditation, aromatherapy, massage, or relaxation devices.

Significant current research supports the use of several herbs that have similar properties and calming effects on anxiety disorders as prescription medications, without the side effects. American ginseng contains ginsenosides that is believed to reduce stress and anxiety by reducing blood flow to the brain. Side effects have only been observed when excessive amounts have used. Kava is another herb that has been used for centuries to treat anxiety. Kavalactones, the active ingredient in Kava is believed to work by modifying action of neurotransmitters, creating a calming effect. Side effects of Kava are reported with high doses. Valerian, a herb that has been used for over 1,000 years as a calming sleep aid has been proven to be effective in treating anxiety, stress-related headaches, tension and insomnia. Unlike prescription sedatives it does not interfere with sleep cycles. Side effects have been observed with over consumption or when used in combination with prescription tranquilizers.

Other less "clinically" studied herbs that have been reported to have calming effects on the nervous system include Lavender, an aromatic herb that is used internally, externally and in aromatherapy, Skullcap/Virginian, used as a sedative and digestive aid, Chamomile, used as a central nervous system sedative, Lemon Balm, also sedating and will relieve indigestion, and Passionflower, used for chronic stress relief, anxiety and insomnia. Aromatherapy uses essential oils of flowers, plants, and herbs to promote healing and well being. Essential oils of Clary Sage, Lavender, Melissa, Rose, and Ylang-Ylang are used to relieve stress in bath oils and massage oils. Combining essentials oils with therapeutic massage produces deep relation that can alleviate stress and anxiety for days.

Nutritional interventions that can reduce anxiety include reducing sugar, food additives, and caffeine consumption, and increasing omega-3 EFA's, vitamins C and B-complex, vitamin E, pantothenic acid, and minerals such as calcium, magnesium, potassium, selenium, and zinc. A natural diet with whole grains, vegetables, fruits and fish can supply many of the basic nutrients needed for proper adrenal gland and nervous system function, however, additional supplementation may also be needed. In addition to stress, environmental toxins like copper deplete necessary vitamins and minerals from the body.

Yoga, a practice that uses therapeutic exercise and meditation has been shown to treat stress and anxiety disorders such as OCD. Meditation produces a condition known as blanking-out. This state is responsible for reducing levels of stress-related chemicals like adrenaline and cortisol, reducing heart rate and blood pressure. Blanking out can be produced through meditation or through devices like a floatation chamber. The floatation chamber eliminates all outside stimuli from an individual allowing them to achieve a deep meditative state that produces relaxation and stress relief for days.

Hypnotherapy utilizes controlled "Blanking-out." It has been used for thousands of years to cure a variety of physical and mental disorders. The therapy works largely due to the patient believing in the "powers" of the hypnotherapist. Before the use of anesthesia in medical operations, hypnotherapy was widely used to relax and even sedate patients. Today it continues to have many therapeutic benefits not only in relaxing the patient, but also in overcoming specific phobias.

Holistic Mental Health for Anxiety & Stress Specific Recommendations:

In treating anxiety, its severity needs to first be determined. If the anxiety is mild counseling and psychotherapy with nutritional intervention may produce desired results without the use of prescription medications. If the condition is interfering with daily functioning such as not allowing the individual to leave the house, or function at school or work, a combination of therapies may be required. However, due to the severity of the side effects of most antidepressant medications treatment should proceed from the least precarious. Anti-anxiety medications may also not uncover the cause of the disorder, but just sedate the individual. If the disorder is due to a possible chemical imbalance, diet and nutritional interventions could correct the imbalance. The following is recommended:

- Restrict sugar, processed foods, and caffeine from the diet.
- Eat a diet rich in organic foods such as whole grains, vegetables, fruits and fish.
- Take a multi-vitamin/mineral daily with additional vitamin C (2-3,000 mg, per day) B-Complex (100 mg 2 times per day), vitamin E (400-800 IU's per day), calcium (1,200-1,500 mg, per day), magnesium (600-800 mg, per day) selenium (75-100 mcg, per day), zinc (30-40 mg, per day).
- Additional essential fatty acids should be taken by eating cold water fish (salmon, tuna) or taking an Alpha-linolenic acid supplement.
- Take American ginseng (1 gram per day) or Kava kava (60 to 120 mg, per day).
- If stress or anxiety is causing insomnia try Valerian an hour before bedtime (50 to 150 mg).
- Use aromatherapy at home by using scented oils, bath oils or soaps such as Lavender, Melissa or Rose.
- Get a therapeutic massage with essential oils such as Clary sage, Lavender, Melissa, Rose, or Ylang-Ylang.
- Try yoga or spend time each day in meditation.
- See a certified hypnotherapist.

- Counseling intervention may be needed to determine if psychotherapy will be helpful if the anxiety disorder is a specific phobia,

- Posttraumatic Stress Disorder, or Obsessive-Compulsive Disorder.

- If a combination of several of the non-meditative approaches are not working after a number of months more serious underlying causes may be at work. Consultation with a holistic physician is recommended.

Treatment for medical conditions should always be conducted by your healthcare professional. According to the FDA only physicians are allowed to prescribe medications, and the suggestions in this book are for dietary changes and/or supplements only.

*"Self-discipline is when
conscience tells you to do something,
and you don't talk back."*
~ *W. K. Hope*

*"Try?
Do, or do not,
there is no try."*
~ *Yoda*

CHAPTER IV:
ATTENTION-DEFICIT/HYPERACTIVITY
DISORDER

Attention-Deficit/Hyperactivity Disorder (ADHD) is considered the most common childhood neurobehavioral disorder of school-aged children today. And, it is the most controversial disorder also. Controversial when we check beyond mainstream allopathic diagnosis and treatment. Today there are many physicians, psychiatrists and psychologists that question whether such a disorder even exists. And, they refuse to recommend psycho-stimulate medication for the "disorder's" symptoms, but seek alternative therapies.

According to the DSM-IV, children with ADHD display problematic behaviors at home and 80 percent are believed to display academic performance problems. Estimates range between 4 to 12 percent of school children have the disorder [1]. Latest statistics from the CDC report that 4.7 million children, including 9.5% of boys and 5.9 % of girls have been diagnosed with the disorder [2]. Children that are diagnosed with ADHD usually are put on psycho-stimulate medication with what seems to be little concern of short-term or long-term side effects.

Of the five million children today with ADHD over two million take Ritalin (methylphenidate) with sometimes only cursory medical/professional diagnosis of the disorder [3, 4, 5]. The medical community appears to be more concern with controlling the student's behavior with drugs rather than trying to determine a cause of the condition. However, there are a number of theories today that address the cause and treatment of the condition without the use of potentially harmful medications.

CLASSIFICATION of ADHD

The Diagnostic and Statistical Manual of Mental Disorders (DSM-IV) currently recognizes three subtypes of ADHD: combined type; predominantly hyperactive-impulsive type; and predominantly inattentive type. The combined and predominantly hyperactive-impulsive sub-types make up the majority (about two-thirds) of individuals with the disorder.

These are the students we typically think of when we talk about ADHD. However, the remaining third fall into the predominantly inattentive subtype. These individuals are often commonly referred to as having simply ADD or Attention Deficit Disorder. While each of the subtypes has certain diagnostic criterion in common (e.g., symptoms will have been present prior to age seven, symptoms are present in two or more settings, and evidence of clinically significant impairment in social, academic or occupational functioning), they are distinguished by their own unique diagnostic criteria or symptoms [6].

Although not all children diagnosed with ADHD are hyperactive, those who are stand out. They tend to be overly restless and impulsive and, to a greater degree and get in more situations than their non-hyperactive peers. Their inability to control their behavior and frequent emotional outbursts is pronounced. It's been said of these individuals that they are, "everywhere at once and nowhere very long." They are often out of their seats, always touching something or someone, rarely satisfied and seldom sticking with a single project. In order for a student to be diagnosed with ADHD, predominantly hyperactive-impulsive type, six or more of the following symptoms will have persisted for at least six months to a degree that is maladaptive and inconsistent with developmental level:

Hyperactivity:

- Fidgets with hands or feet or squirms in seat.
- Often leaves seat in classroom or in other situations in which remaining seated is expected.
- Often runs about or climbs excessively in situations in which it is

inappropriate (in adolescents or adults, may be limited to subjective feelings of restlessness).

- Often has difficulty playing or engaging in leisure activities quietly.
- Is often "on the go" or often acts as if "driven by a motor."
- Often talks excessively.

Impulsivity:

- Often blurts out answers before questions have been completed.
- Often has difficulty awaiting turn.
- Often interrupts or intrudes on others (e.g., butts into conversations or games).

The student diagnosed with ADHD, predominantly inattentive type, or ADD, struggles with inattention but not hyperactivity or impulsiveness. In fact, they have often been described as lethargic and sluggish, daydreamers. They are slow in completing tasks and can seem lost in their own thoughts. Research suggests that students with predominantly inattentive type are at a higher risk for academic failure and have a higher rate of learning problems than the hyperactive-impulsive group and may develop emotional problems related to depression, anxiety and poor self-concept more readily than their hyperactive counterparts. In order for a student to be diagnosed with ADD, six or more of the following symptoms will have persisted for at least six months to a degree that is maladaptive and inconsistent with developmental level:

- Often fails to give close attention to details or makes careless mistakes in schoolwork, work, or other activities.
- Often has difficulty sustaining attention in tasks or play activities.
- Often does not seem to listen when spoken to directly.
- Often does not follow through on instructions and fails to finish schoolwork, chores, or duties in the workplace (not due to oppositional behavior or failure to understand instructions).
- Often has difficulty organizing tasks and activities.
- Often avoids, dislikes, or is reluctant to engage in tasks that require sustained mental effort (such as schoolwork or homework).
- Often looses things necessary for tasks or activities.

- Is often easily distracted by extraneous stimuli.

- Is often forgetful in daily activities.

The student diagnosed with ADHD, combined type, will have met the criteria for both the hyperactive-impulsive type and the inattentive type for at least six months and to a degree that is maladaptive and inconsistent with developmental level [7].

Diagnosis of ADHD

The American Academy of Pediatrics (AAP) calls ADHD the most common childhood neurobehavioral disorder, estimating that between 4 and 12 percent of all school-age children may have the condition [8]. Not surprisingly, the AAP questions the possible over-diagnosis of ADHD.

In their May, 2000 issue of *Pediatrics* the AAP calls for stricter guidelines for primary care physicians diagnosing ADHD in children age 6 to 12 years-old. These guidelines include: using the DSM-IV criteria, with symptoms being present in two or more settings, the symptoms adversely affecting the child's academic or social functioning for at least six months, the assessment should include information from parents as well as classroom teachers or other school professionals, and the evaluation of ADHD should also include an assessment for co-existing conditions such as learning or language problems [9].

The AAP appears to be concerned that far too many physicians will place a child on psychostimulate medication with little or no assessment of the condition. Often they speak only to the parents or give the child a quick in-office physical before writing a prescription for Ritalin [10, 11, 12, 13].

The National Association of School Psychologists (NASP) in their text *Best Practices in School Psychology* (1995), outlines specific criteria children must meet in order to be diagnosed with ADHD [14]. This criteria not only includes DSM-IV guidelines but meets federal requrements for evaluating a child to qualify for educational services under the Individuals with Disabilities Education Act (IDEA).

Therefore, school psychologists are often faced with the task of reconciling confused communication among parents (who believe something is not right with their child), school personnel (who have strict federal guidelines in order service students with special needs) and medical personnel (that label children ADHD and prescribe medications without any testing) [15].

Causes of ADHD

The medical community appears to down play any one deciding factor that would cause ADHD, and would rather list several factors that may contribute to the condition. K. S.. Berger, author of *The Developing Person Through the Life Span.* (1998), indicates current research lists factors such as genetics, prenatal damage from teratogens, or postnatal damage, such as from lead poisoning or head trauma as the cause of ADHD [16].

Genetics

Russell Barkley, Ph.D. [17] author of several books on ADHD such as *Taking Charge of ADHD,* (1995) cites recent research indicating that the areas of the brain in children with ADHD are reduced in size when compared with children without the disorder. Possible causes for the reduction could be polygenetic in nature. Specifically genes that dictate the way the brain uses a neurotransmitter called the dopamine receptor are thought to be mutated in children with ADHD. Other theories include prenatal alcohol consumption, fatty acid deficiency, faulty glucose metabolism, and thyroid abnormalities as possible causes of ADHD [18].

Researchers from the National Institute of Mental Health report a link between a dopamine receptor and a variation of a gene controlling that receptor. In the study children with ADHD were more likely to have a variation of the DRD4 gene, that helps produce dopamine in the brain. However, not all the children in the study with ADHD had the DRD4 variation, and all the children with ADHD had taken stimulate medication [19].

Thyroid Dysfunction

A variety of recent observations have led investigators to conclude there is a relationship between thyroid dysfunction and ADHD. It has been observed that up to 70 percent of all children with a condition known as "generalized thyroid resistance" also demonstrate ADHD symptoms. Patients with thyroid resistance suffer from altered glucose uptake by cells, a feature that we now know impairs brain metabolism. Altered glucose uptake is linked to ADHD if that diminished brain activity happens to be in the brain regions responsible for our ability to pay attention and control our behavior.

Thyroid dysfunction may be caused by synthetic chemicals like PCBs, phenols, thiols, and excessive histamines. A fatty acid deficiency is also related to thyroid dysfunction. A large portion of the brain is composed of fats, called phospholipids that are derived from essential fatty acids. A number of studies have identified an essential fatty acid (EFA) deficiency in many hyperactive children. For example, a 1995 study published in *The American Journal of Clinical Nutrition* showed a correlation between low omega-3 blood levels and ADHD in young boys. EFAs play important roles in neurotransmitter function in communication of neurotransmitters and in proper nerve cell development [20].

Diet: Sugar Metabolism

Sugar appears to be highly controversial regarding its effect on children and the possibility of it causing ADHD. Depending on which study you read, you can be thoroughly confused as to its relation to children's behavior. Bricklin, in *The Practical Encyclopedia of Natural Healing* (1983) reports of a 5-year study by Dr. William Crook, a pediatrician whom had been treating hyperactive children for 25 years. In his study he interview parents of 182 hyperactive children and found the great majority of the children were adversely affected by their diet. He found their hyperactivity was definitely related to specific foods the worst offender being sugar.

Another study by the New York Institute of Child Development in New York City involved 265 hyperactive children. They found that 74 percent of the children had an inability to properly digest and assimilate sugar and other refined carbohydrates [21]. A study conducted by the National Institute of Mental Health showed that the rate at which the brain uses glucose, its main energy source, is lower with subjects with ADHD than with subjects without ADHD [22].

Dr. Jay Lombard in his *The Brain Wellness Plan* (1997) treatment for ADHD first recommends assessing the patient with ADHD for both reactivity to sugar intake and potential glucose intolerance [23].

Mary Block, M.D., in *No More Ritalin, Treating ADHD Without Drugs* (1996) explains how reactive hypoglycemia and adrenaline levels are related. Dr. Block states when we have too little glucose in our body (blood sugar) the body releases a backup reserve called epinephrine or adrenaline. Adrenaline is a hormone that gives the body an energy surge. The body goes into hypoglycemia (low blood sugar) by either not eating enough or paradoxically by eating too much sugar. People with reactive hypoglycemia may have a metabolism problem that cause the over secretion of adrenaline.

Dr. Block cites a Yale study that tested the effects of sugar on blood glucose and adrenaline levels. The study showed the adrenaline levels of children were ten times higher than normal up to five hours after ingesting the sugar. She explains that many studies that show a poor relationship between sugar intake and behavior are usually flawed and poorly conducted. She also makes the point if any medical professionals questions the effect sugar has on behavior they should talk to a parent or teacher around Halloween [24].

By using PET scans of the brain scientists are able to visually observe the amount of glucose certain areas of the brain uses. In examining the brains of people with ADHD, there are certain areas of the brain that show decreased use of glucose and diminished brain metabolism. Scientists are currently searching for the cause of this decreased glucose metabolism in people with ADHD.

A questionable study concerning the effects of sugar and behavior is used as the basis to discount the relationship by Dr. Isadore Rosenfeld in his book *Doctor What Should I Eat?* (1995). He uses the study of 48 hyperactive children (25 who were of pre-school age) who were fed diets high in sugar and observed for three weeks for changes in behavior. Stating that no changes were noted, he recommends that parents need not pay attention to their child's sugar intake [25].

Two major questions occur with the study he quotes. First, the number of children in the study appears far too small, the 25 pre-school children should not have been diagnosed with ADHD. DSM-IV criteria, AAP, and NASP all recommend not labeling any children under the age of 6 with ADHD, leaving 23 children in the study. Secondly, if the children are already ADHD and may be having poor reactions to sugar how could there be much of a noticeable change in behavior? Should they have tried eliminating sugars altogether from a control group of ADHD children (over 6 years old) and measure any change in behavior for a better determination of a relationship? [25, 26, 27]

Fetal Alcohol Syndrome

Another observed neurodevelopment disorder that leads to ADHD symptoms has been associated with fetal alcohol syndrome (FAS). FAS is caused by over consumption of alcohol during pregnancy, and children with FAS are characterized with low birth weight, an impaired intellect, and certain physical defects. Children born with FAS show the same hyperactivity, low impulse control, and inability to pay attention as those children diagnosed with ADHD [28].

Food Additives

In the 1970's Ben Feingold, M.D., developed one of the first natural approaches to treating hyperactivity. He was a pediatrician who taught at Northwestern University and a pioneer in the fields of allergy and immunology. He also served as Chief of Allergies at the *Kaiser Permanente Medical Center* in San Francisco.

According to Dr. Feingold many hyperactive children are sensitive to naturally occurring salicylates and phenolic compounds. Salicylates are used as food preservatives and in the production of aspirin. Dr. Feingold determined that food additives induce hyperactivity after researching over 1,200 cases where additives were linked to behavior disorders. Dr. Feingold believes that salicylates, artificial colors, and artificial flavors in the diet are responsible for hyperactivity in children [29].

Dr. Weintraub reports as far back as 1940 there have been reports of sensitivities to food dyes, aspirin, and naturally occurring salicylate substances found in fruits and vegetables. Dr. Weintraub cites other studies in support of Dr. Feingold's theory [28]. A study published in *Lancet* (1985) found that 82 percent of a large group of hyperactive children responded positively to a hypoallergenic elimination diet. While on the diet many of the children's behavior became normal [30]. The most commonly provoking substances were artificial food colors and preservatives.

Dr. Carl Pfeiffer M.D. recommends a natural diet for hyperactive children based on the belief that food additives, artificial colors, flavors and preservatives causes hyperactivity. Another study in support of Dr. Feingold's theories, was a study of 76 hyperactive children. When placed on a restricted diet devoid of additives 62 of the children improved and 21 realized normal behavior [31].

Dr. Weintraub discusses a recent study conducted at the Royal Children's Hospital, University of Melbourne, Australia of 200 hyperactive children. In a six week trial, the children were placed on a diet free of all synthetic foods. The parents of 150 children reported significant behavioral improvements, however, they noted when artificial colors were added back into their diets their behavior worsened. The more food coloring they consumed, the longer the undesirable behavior lasted [32].

A 1994 study at the North Shore Hospital-Cornell Medical Center found that by eliminating reactive foods such as those with food additives and artificial colors the ADHD symptoms of irritability, restlessness, sleep disturbances and other negative behaviors were reduced [33].

In a 2008 article, professor of pediatrics from the University of Sydney, Andrew Kemp, MD, states that dietary modifications should be part of the standard treatment for ADHD. Kemp cited a recent controlled trial showing an increase in hyperactivity among children that had not been diagnosed with ADHD that were fed a diet high in food colorings and the preservative sodium benzoate. He noted that of 22 studies conducted between 1975 and 1994, 16 found dietary modification to have a positive impact on some children with

ADHD. Just as not all children respond to psycho-stimulate medication, he suggested that dietary modification has been shown to have more positive benefits than behavioral therapy, yet it had been widely dismissed by the medical profession as an alternative treatment for ADHD. Kemp states "in view of the relatively harmless intervention of eliminating colorings and preservatives, and the large number of children taking drugs for hyperactivity, it might be proposed that an appropriately supervised and evaluated trial of eliminating colorings and preservatives should be part of standard treatment for children" [34].

Psychostimulate Medication

Peter Breggin, MD, is a psychiatrist that has been specializing in ADHD treatment for over 30 years. In his books, *Talking Back to Ritalin,* (2001), and *The Ritalin Fact Book, What Your Doctor Won't Tell You about Stimulant Drugs,* (2002) he contends that ADHD is a disorder that was fabricated by the pharmaceutical companies in order to sell their drugs. He refutes the medical evidence that ADHD is a neurological disorder by pointing out that the research that showed reduced attention centers in ADHD children was flawed.

At the National Institute of Mental Health's Conference on ADHD (1998) Dr. Breggin was invited to speak and was one of the few critics of conventional psycho-stimulate therapy for ADHD. At that conference he pointed out that the studies on brain atrophy of ADHD children involved children that had already been on psycho-stimulate medication. And, that previous studies have shown that psycho-stimulate medications in fact, causes brain atrophy. That conference, that had 30 national experts on ADHD concluded that there is currently no conclusive evidence that suggests that ADHD is a medical disorder.

In his books Dr. Breggin presents clinical studies that show that there are little long-term educational benefits in using psycho-stimulates. And, he elaborates on the many significant harmful effects of the drugs. Dr. Breggin has also been involved several individual and class-action suits as an expert witness against the pharmaceutical companies over wrongful deaths and ill effects from the drugs prescribed for ADHD [35].

Is ADHD a Disorder?

Just as Dr. Breggin above does not believe ADHD is a "disorder," David Stein, Ph.D. also questions if ADHD is a medical disorder at all. He states that there is little scientific evidence to support that it is a medical condition. Dr.

Stein suggests that the environment a child is brought up in is the primary reason for ADHD behavior. In his book, *Ritalin Is Not The Answer* (1999), he contends lack of discipline in the home or in the classroom is the main cause of ADHD. He believes by setting consistent boundaries with behavior control interventions, ADHD symptoms can be eliminated [36].

In my 25 years as an educator and school psychologist, I would strongly agree with Dr. Breggin and Dr. Stein. Granted, I have observed and worked with many students that exhibit hyperactivity and inattention in the classroom, but I question whether they have a "disorder" or just disinterest in school. These same children that cannot concentrate in the classroom, can play video games for hours on end at home, have no problem watching their favorite TV shows or a movie for two hours at a time.

Therefore, is ADHD an inattention problem or just an interest problem? How can they turn their inattention, their ADHD, on and off at will? These same students that have an inattention problem in one class don't exhibit any problems in another class they are interested in or one that they like the teacher in. Again, they are able to turn their ADHD on and off at will. Many students do exhibit physical hyperactivity (high degrees of activity like running, jumping, tapping or shaking body parts) but is that not diet related? If their main fuel is sugar why wouldn't they exhibit such activity? If an adult consumes and excessive amount of caffeine wouldn't they exhibit nervousness and hyperactivity also? I do not believe a disorder, certainly not a "medical" disorder can be turned on and off at will.

Allopathic Treatment:

Allopathic treatment for ADHD consistent primarily of prescribing psycho-stimulants to control the child's behavior. Physicians prescribe a psychic-stimulant like Ritalin, Concerta or Adderall usually starting in a small dose (5 or 10 mg) and increase it monthly based on a reduction of the ADHD symptoms. Side-effects are monitored and medications are often switched if side-effects are too severe or if there is no noticeable difference in the child's behavior.

Additional medications may also be prescribed like Trazadone, to help the child sleep at night, or an anti-anxiety medication if they develop twitches or tics (Paxil, Wellbutrin, Klonopin). Occasionally the ups and downs of the medications causes the child to hallucinate or have "mood swings" and they are then diagnosed with Bipolar Disorder (becoming a very popular childhood diagnosis) and anti-psychotic medication is prescribed (like Depakote or Zyprexa). Table 4-1 describes the most common medications used for ADHD.

Table 4-1
Summary of Allopathic Treatment for ADHD [37, 38, 39]:

Drug: *(brand name)*	*Acting mechanism:*	*Possible side effects:*
Methylphenidate hydrochloride *(Ritalin, Ritalin XR, Concerta, Daytrana),* **Dexmethylphen-idate hydrochloride** *(Focalin)*	Central nervous system stimulate that activates the brainstem arousal system and cerebral cortex and thereby decreases motor restlessness, increases attention span, and improves concentration. Increases the production of neuro-transmitter (dopamine).	Common include; insomnia, nervousness, loss of appetite, abdominal pain, weight loss, and abnormally fast heartbeat. Less common may include; abdominal pain, abnormal heartbeat, abnormal muscular movements, blood pressure changes, dizziness, drowsiness, fever, hair loss, headache, hives, joint pain, nausea, palpitations, skin inflammation, skin rash, Tourette's syndrome, and psychotic reactions.
***d*-amphetamine and amphetamine mixture** *(Adderall, Adderall XR)*	Blocks the reuptake of neurotransmitters, thereby prolonging their actions and slows down metabolism.	Irritability, nervousness, insomnia, euphoria, dry mouth, rapid heartbeat, dizziness, reduced alertness, blurred vision, headache, diarrhea or constipation, appetite loss, nausea, weight loss, seizures, irregular heartbeat, habit forming.

Pemoline *(Cylert)*	Similar operating mechanism to Adderall but with less stimulate effects, and is less abusive.	Insomnia, irritability, loss of appetitive, weight loss, depression, dizziness, headache, drowsiness, stomach ache, nausea, skin rash, irregular heartbeat, muscle twitches, hallucinations, liver damage.
Dextroamphetamine *(Dexedrine)*	CNS stimulant that decreases motor restlessness, increases attention.	Irritability, nervousness, insomnia, euphoria, dry mouth, rapid heartbeat, dizziness, reduced alertness, blurred vision, headache, diarrhea or constipation, appetite loss, nausea, weight loss, seizures, irregular heartbeat, habit forming.
Methamphetamine *(Desoxyn)*	CNS stimulant that decreases motor restlessness, increases attention.	Irritability, nervousness, insomnia, euphoria, dry mouth, rapid heartbeat, dizziness, reduced alertness, blurred vision, headache, diarrhea or constipation, appetite loss, nausea, weight loss, seizures, irregular heartbeat, habit forming.
Desipramine *(Norpramin)*	A secondary tricyclic antidepressant that blocks norepinephrine a neuro-transmitter.	Sedation, dry mouth, urinary hesitation, constipation, dizziness. Less common; psychoses, suicidal behavior. Not FDA approved for children.
Atomoxetine *(Strattera)*	Blocks neurotransmitters function increasing attention.	Appetitive loss, mood swings, nausea, vomiting, dizziness, tiredness, insomnia, dry mouth, constipation, impotence.

Imipramine hydrochoride *(Tofranil)*	A tricyclic antidepressant that blocks serotonin a neuro-transmitter.	Sedation, dry mouth, urinary hesitation, constipation, dizziness. Less common; psychoses, suicidal behavior.
Lisdexamfetamine dimesylate *(Vyvanse)*	CNS stimulant that decreases motor restlessness, increases attention.	Appetitive loss, nausea, vomiting, irritability, insomnia, mania, abnormal thoughts/behavior, growth suppression, Tourette's syndrome.

Effects of Psycho-stimulate Medications:

Table 4-1 illustrates side effects of psycho-stimulates can range from mild to life threatening. The medical community appears to dismiss the growth suppression side effect of psycho-stimulates, however when appetite loss and weight loss are a common side effect, and most children take ADHD medications during their developmental years, it would make sense that their growth rates would be suppressed. A study by James Swanson, PhD, director of the Child Development Center at the University of California supported the claim that psycho-stimulate drugs like Ritalin does in fact, stunts children's growth. His study claims that after three years on drugs like Ritalin children are an inch shorter, and 4.4 pounds lighter than their peers [40].

In 2006 an advisory panel urged the FDA to placed warnings on all psycho-stimulate drugs used to treat ADHD due to the potential risk of heart attacks, strokes and sudden death. The panel cited studies that showed an elevated occurrence of heart attacks and strokes in adults taking ADHD drugs. Children on the drugs showed a higher-than-expected number of strokes. In the adult study, 732 heart attacks were observed when only 218 were expected, and 401 strokes occurred where 164 were expected. In a study of children and adolescents taking ADHD drugs 49 cases of heart attacks occurred when 12 were expected. The FDA also received reports of 20 sudden deaths of children taking Adderall, one of the more popular ADHD drugs. Those reports prompted the Canadian government to order Adderall off the shelves in February, 2006 [41].

In February, 2007, the FDA did require that medications used to treat ADHD be accompanied by information warning about the use of these drugs in patients with heart problems [42]. The American Heart Association called for all children and teens taking stimulate medication for ADHD to be screened for hidden heart problems in April, 2008. The AHA recommended that in addition to a careful medical history and physical examination, and electrocardiogram (ECG) be performed prior to starting any child or adolescent on stimulant medications. The AMA is concerned that as many as 2 percent of children in the U.S. have undiagnosed heart problems that could be identified by ECG screening. They also called for periodic cardiac evaluations by patients taking ADHD drugs. Their guideline states that blood pressure and pulse rates should be evaluated during routine follow-up visits every one to three months [43].

The FDA did recommend discontinuing the use of Cylert, and any generic versions of the drug (pemoline). Although the drug did come with warnings of liver failure as a side effect of its use, the FDA now believes that the risk of liver failure outweighs any benefits of the drug. 13 reported cases of liver failure resulting in death occurred due to use of the drug. The FDA reported that although 13 isn't a large number during the drug's use in the past 20 years, the rate of failure was still 10 to 25 times greater when using the drug. The manufacturer of the drug, Abbott did discontinue the sale of Cylert in 2006 citing financial reasons for its being withdrawn from the market [44].

FDA officials are requiring (as of January, 2009) new labeling on ADHD drugs including Ritalin LA, Concerta, Adderall XR, Focalin XR, Medadate CD, Daytrana, and Strattera, of warning of possible psychiatric side effects. FDA researchers identified more than 350 separate incidences of hallucinations and other psychotic episodes among children taking stimulants to treat ADHD. Nearly half of the cases reported involved children under the age of 11, and 9 out of 10 of the cases, the children had no reported history of psychiatric events. The most common hallucinations involved insects, worms or snakes crawling on or around the children and teens taking the drugs [45].

Children on ADHD drugs are more likely abuse alcohol as teenagers. A Pittsburgh ADHD longitudinal study of 364 children found that more than twice as many had problems wit alcohol than the norm. The study found that 14 percent of the children in their late teen years developed alcohol abuse problems compared to 5 percent of their peers that were not labeled with ADHD or on ADHD drugs. Before age 15 children with ADHD did not abuse alcohol any more than other children [46].

Naturopathic Treatment

There are many factors that are leading a number of doctors to question the diagnosis of ADHD. Such as the significant side-effects of the medications prescribed to children diagnosed with ADHD. There is the question of little long-term improvement academically of students on these medications. And there is the question of the criteria that actually diagnoses ADHD.

When looking into the DSM-IV criteria for ADHD many are struck with the realization that 9 out of 10 children could be diagnosed with the "disorder." It appears that many normal childhood behaviors like: *"fails to finish schoolwork or chores," "often dislikes and avoids homework!"* or, *"has difficulty awaiting turn,"* are used to determine if a child has ADHD. Then there is the realization that psycho-stimulates do not cure the cause of the behaviors, but merely supply the patient with a bandage (life-long?) for the disorder. However, many naturopathic therapies may in fact cure the "disorder."

A recent clinical study that measured the effectiveness of nutritional interventions compared to traditional psycho-stimulant treatment reported: "these findings support the effectiveness of food supplement treatment in improving attention and self-control in children with ADHD and suggest food supplement treatment of ADHD may be of equal efficacy to Ritalin treatment." [47]

Since Dr. Feingold pioneered his theories of diet-related causes for hyperactive behavior there have been several variations in support of a more natural diet as a cure. Dr. Feingold's diet has been called an elimination diet due to the process he recommends of first eliminating all foods that contain natural and synthetic salicylates. Natural salicylates include fruits and vegetables such as almonds, apples, apricots, berries, cherries, grapes, raisins, oranges, peaches, plums, prunes, strawberries, pickles, tomatoes, cucumbers and vinegar.

Synthetic salicylates include all foods that contain artificial colors and artificial flavors, such as benzoic acid, BHA, BHT, MSG, butylene glycol, potassium bisulfate, potassium and sodium nitrate, sulfites, and tartrazines. Once a child's behavior is normalized, which may take four to six weeks, food items may slowly reintroduced into their diet and monitored for their effect on the child's behavior [48].

Frank Lawlis, Ph.D. in his book *The ADD Answer: How to Help Your Child Now,* expands Dr. Feingold's diet and gives specific diet recommendations for the child with ADHD. He recommends the entire family follow such a diet to give the child support, as the diet can be very restrictive (see table 4-2). Dr. Lawlis states that foods that have a negative impact on children's health include: artificial colors and preservatives, processed milk and milk products, wheat products (not whole grains), sugar, oranges, grapefruits, eggs, and MSG. He also recommends a diet rich in calcium, magnesium, zinc (important in proper neurotransmitter function), vitamins C and B_6

(important in immune system and metabolism function), B$_{12}$ (increases energy, lessens anxiety, increases concentration), fish oil (contains DHA important in brain health), protein (stimulates mental alertness), pycnogenol or grape seed extract (two herbs that increase blood flow in the brain) and probiotic (helps restore healthy bacteria in the intestines).

Dr. Lawlis warns that medications used for ADHD can cause severe side-effects such as psychosis, including manic and schizophrenic episodes. And often when such side-effects occur physicians do not stop medicating, they prescribe more drugs, diagnosing the child with depression or antisocial personality disorder, and they treat the child with antidepressants, mood stabilizers or narcoleptics. It is not unusual for children to be taking as many as five different medications that cause a host of side-effects. He states "meds upon meds is madness upon madness" [49].

Bricklin describes natural therapy of increased protein in the diet to increase serotonin, which has a calming effect on children with hyperactivity. He also recommends large amounts of B vitamins, with emphasis on B$_6$ (pyridoxine), vitamin C, and essential fatty acids (EFA's) [50]. Similar dietary recommendations have been made by Pfeiffer (1987) [51], Weintraub (1997) [52], Mindell (1994) [53], Block (1996) [54], Lombard and Germano (1997) [55], Tenney (1997) [56], and Nambudripad (1999) [57].

Dr. Weintraub in addition, recommends an iron and zinc deficiency and imbalances of sodium-potassium, phosphorus or copper as contributing factors to ADHD. Along with increasing mineral supplementation Dr. Weintraud suggests herbal supplements such as alfalfa, astragalus, borage, catnip, chamomile, ginger root, gotu kola, kava kava, kelp lavender, lemon balm, passionflower, red clover, rosemary, skullcap, Siberian ginseng, St. John's wort, and valerian as possible herbs that have positive effects of reducing hyperactivity [58].

Tenney recommends natural therapy of keeping the bowels clean to avoid the accumulation of toxins and hair analysis to determine if there are any heavy metal poisoning in the body. In addition to B-complex and vitamin C, she recommends vitamin A to help protect against allergies, and multi-minerals with extra calcium, magnesium, selenium and zinc. Specific herbs she recommends for ADHD include black walnut (kills parasites), burdock (cleans blood), catnip (relaxes), dandelion (cleans liver), gotu kola (brain food), lobelia, red clover, and skullcap (builds nerves) [59].

Salaman cites research that used high doses of vitamin B6 (pyridoxine) to control hyperactivity. In the study, high doses of B6 were given to hyperactive children for seven weeks followed by seven weeks of Ritalin, and seven weeks of a placebo. The high dose of B6 proved to be the most effective treatment, where it raised the blood serotonin level and Ritalin did not. Salaman also recommends EFA supplementation of 1,000 to 1,500 mg capsules of evening primrose in the morning and evening. She notes some children respond better if the evening primrose oil is rubbed into their skin, as quite often children with hyperactivity may have poor intestinal tract absorption [60].

Table 4-2
Recommended Diet for ADHD [13, 49]:

Food Group:	Rec. Servings:	Examples of Foods:
Protein	2	Lean meats, poultry, fish, eggs, legumes, tofu.
Fruits & Vegetables	5	Any fruits and vegetables except: apples, apricots, berries, cherries, grapes, raisins, oranges, peaches, plums, prunes, strawberries, pickles, tomatoes. cucumbers and vinegar.
Milk substitutes	3	Rice milk or soy milk products, yogurt, cottage cheese. Sugar-free ice cream or ice milk. Cheesecake.
Whole grains	4	Whole wheat grains and pastas, rice.
Fats	Use sparingly	Olive oil, flaxseed oil, natural peanut butter, nuts (except almonds).

Conclusions:

ADHD continues to be the most controversial mental disorder. Concerned with the harmful side effects of psycho-stimulants many healthcare professionals are seeking alternative treatments. A primary philosophical issue of the ADHD treatment is should we chemically control our children? Should 5 or 6 year old boys be chemically controlled by psycho-stimulate medication for acting like little boys?

Current research does support natural treatment for ADHD, a disorder that is considered an unnatural reaction to environmental factors (if in fact such a disorder exists). There appears to be substantial evidence to support dietary factors that cause ADHD behaviors that includes sugar consumption, reaction to food additives, faulty glucose metabolism (sugar consumption), and fatty acid deficiency. Parents do in fact have a choice when it comes to treatment for their children. They no longer have to place their child on potentially harmful psycho-stimulate medications. Or, possibly risk a life long pattern of drug dependence for their children.

Medications such as Ritalin, Adderall, Concerta, Strattera, Cylert, Dexedrine, Tofranil, and Norpramin have side effects that range from mild (dry mouth, nausea, headaches, dizziness, constipation, irritability) to serious (anorexia, insomnia, weight loss, depression, palpitations, blurred vision, high blood pressure), to very serious (suppressed growth, liver damage, Tourette's syndrome, psychosis, drug dependence, even death).

The natural approach to treatment of ADHD may require more time and effort by the family when restricting their child's diet, but the benefits of the approach are great. The cause of the child's behavior will have been uncovered and not just covered-up by treating the symptoms with harmful drugs.

Current research involving the use of multi-vitamin and multi-mineral supplements, herbs and eliminating toxins in the diet such as food colorings, additives and heavy metals, all appear to have a dramatic effect on a reducing a child's ADHD symptoms without harmful side effects.

Holistic Mental Health for ADHD
Specific Recommendations:

Based on this research treatment of ADHD should progress from the least harmful course of action, and try to uncover the cause of the condition. Causes of ADHD that can be treated without psychostimulate medications include food allergies, nutrient deficiencies, and diet restriction intervention. Recommended course of treatment:

- An evaluation with a naturopathic physician to determine if a food allergy exists and a dietary evaluation to determine if a nutrient deficiency exists.

- Eliminate all processed foods that contain artificial additives such as aspartame, benzoic acid, BHA, BHT, MSG, butylene glycol, potassium bisulfate, potassium and sodium nitrate, sulfites, and tartrazines from the diet.

- Eliminate natural salicylates such as almonds, apples, apricots, berries, cherries, grapes, raisins, oranges, peaches, plums, prunes, strawberries, pickles, tomatoes, cucumbers and vinegar from the diet.

- Add a vitamin/mineral supplement daily, with extra B-complex (120 to 150 mg, per day), vitamin C (1,000 to 2,000 mg, per day), calcium (1,000 to 1,500 mg, per day), magnesium (300 to 500 mg, per day), zinc (20 to 30 mg, per day) and selenium (100 to 200 mcg, per day), and an EFA supplement containing omega-3 EFAs such as in EPA fish oil capsules, or take evening primrose oil (2,000 to 3,000 mg, per day in two doses).

- Calming herbs such as St. John's wort (see depression chapter), valerian or skullcap (see anxiety chapter) can be tried to reduce symptoms of hyperactivity and irritability.

Treatment for medical conditions should always be conducted by your healthcare professional. According to the FDA only physicians are allowed to prescribe medications, and the suggestions in this book are for dietary changes and/or supplements only.

"Oftentimes it happens we live our lives in chains,
not realizing we have always had the key."
~ The Eagles

"The past does not equal the future."
~ Anthony Robbins

CHAPTER V:
DEPRESSION

Depression on the Rise!

Research indicates that in a given year, at least 17.5 million American adults, 1 in 10, will experience depression. According to the Epidemiological Catchment Area study, 17 percent of all Americans will experience a major depression in their lifetime. People with depression experience severe functional limitations that are often worse than those of patients who suffer from chronic medical illness. Depression results in a 1.8 fold increased risk for physical disability, and a 23 fold increased risk for social disability [1]. There is an estimated one depressed individual for every 5 families.

Depressive illness may even be growing more prevalent in the US. Research has shown that more people are now developing depression at an earlier age. It is estimated between 3 and 6 million Americans under the age of 18 have depressive illness. Experts believe even infants can get depressed if they are neglected, abused or separated from their mothers. Researchers have found that among children aged 12 and younger, between 1 percent and 2 percent are depressed. This percentage jumps during adolescents, when it is thought about 8 percent of boys and 10 percent of girls become depressed. The rate of depression climbs steeply during their teen years, so that by the end of adolescence about twice as many girls as boys are depressed. Ten percent of the people born between 1940 and 1959 have experienced depression by age 25, whereas, only 2.5 percent of the generation born before 1940 have experienced depression [2].

Prevalence rates of depression in children range between 0.4 percent and 2.5 percent and .4 percent and 8.3 percent in adolescents. However, lifetime prevalence rates of Major Depressive Disorder (MDD) in adolescents has been estimated to range between 15 percent to 20 percent, which is comparable to that which is found in adult populations. This may suggest that depression in adults often begins in adolescence. In children, MDD occurs at approximately the same rate in girls and in boys, however, in adolescents the female-to-male ratio is approximately 2:1, similar to that which is found in adults [3].

Latest statistics from the CDC reports that rates of depression is highest among women, baby boomers aged 40 to 59 and non-Hispanic African Americans then in other demographic groups. Older woman are more likely to be depressed and remain depressed longer than men. Only 29 percent of depressed individuals sought medical help, and only 39% of individuals with severe depression contacted a mental health professional. [4].

Early onset MDD and Dysthymic Disorder (DD), a depressive state for two years, are both frequent, familial, and recurrent disorders that are accompanied by other psychiatric disorders, in particular anxiety and disruptive disorders. Both disorders increase the risk for substance abuse, suicidal behavior, and poor psychosocial and functional outcome. MDD increases the risk of bipolar disorder and DD the risk for the development of future MDD episodes [5].

Types of Depressive Illness

The *Diagnostic and Statistical Manual of Mental Disorders-Fourth Edition -Text Revision* (DSM-IV-TR), by the American Psychological Association (APA), classifies depression as one of two subcategories of Mood Disorders. Mood Disorders are divided into Bipolar Disorders that involve the presence of (or history) of Manic Episodes, Mixed Episodes or Hypomanic Episodes, usually accompanied by the presence (or history) of Major Depressive Episodes, and the Depressive Disorders. Depressive Disorders are further categorized into:

Major Depressive Disorder *(MDD):* Characterized by one or more Major Depressive Episodes (i.e., at least 2 weeks of depressed mood or loss of interest accompanied by at least four additional symptoms of depression).

Dysthymic Disorder: Characterized by at least 2 years of depressed mood for more days than not, accompanied by additional depressive symptoms that do not meet the criteria for a Major Depressive Episode.

Depressive Disorder Not Otherwise Specified: Is included for coding disorders with depressive features that do not meet the criteria for Major Depressive Disorder, Dysthymic Disorder, Adjustment Disorder with Depressed Mood, or Adjustment With Mixed Anxiety and Depressed Mood [6].

Symptoms/ Criteria for Major Depressive Episode:

The APA classifies MDD by the following guidelines:

Five (or more) of the following symptoms have been present during the same two week period and represent a change from previous functioning; at least one of the symptoms is either depressed mood or lost of interest in pleasure:

- Depressed mood most of the day, nearly every day, as indicated by either subjective report or observation made by others.

- Markedly diminished interest in pleasure in all, or almost all, activities most of the day, nearly every day.

- Significant weight loss when not dieting or weight gain (change of more than 5% of body weight in a month) or decrease or increase in appetite nearly every day.

- Insomnia or hypersomnia nearly every day.

- Psychomotor agitation or retardation nearly every day.

- Fatigue or loss of energy nearly every day.

- Feelings of worthlessness or excessive or inappropriate guilt (which may be delusional) nearly every day.

- Diminished ability to think or concentrate or indecisiveness, nearly every day.

- Recurrent thoughts of death, recurrent suicidal ideation without a specific plan, or a suicide attempt or a specific plan for committing suicide.

- The symptoms do not meet the criteria for a Mixed Episode.

- The symptoms cause clinically significant distress or impairment in social, occupational, or other important areas of functioning.

- The symptoms are not due to the direct physiological effects of a substance or a general medical condition.

- The symptoms are not better accounted for bereavement, i.e., after the loss of a loved one, the symptoms persist for longer than 2 months or are characterized by marked functional impairment, morbid preoccupation with worthlessness, suicidal ideation, psychotic symptoms, or psychomotor retardation.

Major Depressive Disorder can be specified based on its severity. If criteria are met for the Major Depressive Episode it can be classified as Mild, Moderate, Severe Without Psychotic Features, or Severe With Psychotic Features. The severity is based on the number of criteria symptoms.

Mild Depression is characterized by the presence of only five or six depressive symptoms and either mild disability or the capacity to function normally but with substantial and unusual effort. Episodes that are Severe Without Psychotic Features are characterized by the presence of most of the criteria symptoms and clear-cut, observable disability. Moderate episodes have a severity that is intermediate between mild and severe. Severe With Psychotic Features indicates the presence of either delusions or hallucinations during the current depressive episode [7].

Causes of Depressive Illness:

Brain Chemistry

The American Medical Association's *Essential Guide To Depression* (1998) states that no one knows exactly what causes major depression, however, there are several current theories. One theory is that abnormal activity in the chemistry of the brain gives rise to the illness. In some people the tendency to develop the disorder may be inherited. In others, depression may be linked to abnormal levels of hormones in the body. Or, depression may be the result of a mistimed biological clock. However, to date there have been no definitive biological tests developed that can diagnosis depression [8].

There have been identifiable links between depression and the activities of three main neurotransmitters in the brain: norepinephrine, serotonin, and dopamine. It is believed that these three neurotransmitters are in the brain areas that control activities that go wrong during depression. Each neurotransmitter operates in a pathway that winds through the brain's pleasure centers, the hypothalamus and the limbic system. These regions are responsible for controlling our emotions, physical drives such as appetite, sleep, sexuality, and our reaction to stress.

Norepinephine is also concentrated in parts of the brain linked with fear and memory. Serotonin follows a similar pathway but originates in certain cells that may play a part in agitation and sleep. Dopamine is active in an area of the brain associated with emotions. Between them, these three neurotransmitters travel on pathways reaching many parts of the brain that control activities disrupted by depression and mania [9].

As scientists learned more about the role of neurotransmitters in the brain they were able to put forth theories of how the supply of neurotransmitters could affect a person's mood, and behavior. These theories were based on the fact that antidepressants can ease depression in some people by adjusting the supply of certain neurotransmitters in the brain.

Two types of antidepressants increase the brain's level of norepinephrine. One type known as tricyclic antidepressants prevents the reuptake of norepinephrine. Another type, called monoamine oxidase inhibitors (MAOIs), stops the breakdown of norepinephrine in the synapse of the neurons in the brain. Because both types of antidepressants boost the brain's concentrations of norepinephrine, early theories suggested that too little norepinephrine caused depression, while too much caused mania. However, this theory was questioned when it was found that some depressed people have high levels of norepinephrine, and that some depressed people do not feel better after an antidepressant increases the levels of norepinephrine. When people do respond to antidepressant medication they usually do so after several weeks even though the medication boasts their norepinephrine level immediately [10].

Similar findings have been made with the neurotransmitters serotonin and dopamine. Researchers have low levels of serotonin in some severely depressed people, including some who were suicidal. Therefore some antidepressants work by increasing the levels of serotonin rather than norepinephrine. However, it has also been found that some depressed people have too much serotonin.

Dopamine levels also change during episodes of the illness. Dopamine levels are found to rise during mania and fall during depression. Medication that reduces dopamine levels such as blood pressure medication reserpine, can sometimes cause depression. Depression can also result when physical illnesses such as Parkinson's disease reduces the supply of dopamine in the brain [11].

Neuropeptides may also play a role in depression. Neuropeptides are chemicals in the body that have characteristics of both neurotransmitters and hormones. They work with neurotransmitters to make neurons more or less receptive to the brain's message. One type of neuropeptides is the group of chemicals called endorphins, which control the brain's perception of pain and response to pain. Some people with minor depressive illness have low amounts of some endorphins.

The amino acid called GABA (gamma-amino-butyric acid) another neurotransmitter, also has been linked to depression. GABA helps to control the flow of nerve impulses blocking the release of other neurotransmitters, such as norepinephrine and dopamine. GABA reduces anxiety when released in the body, low levels of GABA have been discovered in some depressed people [12].

Another theory on the cause of depression has to do with the functioning of the neurotransmitter's receptor site. The receptor site is the part of the neurotransmitter that receives a chemical signal from another neuron. If that receptor is not functioning correctly, depression occurs. Some researchers believe that this may explain how an antidepressant works. If an antidepressant increases the amount of a particular neurotransmitter in your brain, your receptors may respond by becoming less sensitive to that neurotransmitter.

Antidepressants alter two types of receptors for norepinephrine. They make these receptors less sensitive or less abundant. If antidepressants do work by changing receptors this adjustment would take time, which also explains why most antidepressants take effect only after about two weeks [13].

Endocrine System Disorders

The functioning of the endocrine system may also be linked to the cause of depression. The endocrine system helps the brain regulate many of the body's activities. It consists of many tiny organs called glands that manufacture hormones and release them into the blood. Hormones control many of the body's physical processes, including sexual development and reaction to stress. Hormones travel through the body where they cause changes to occur. A significant number of depressed people have abnormal amounts of certain hormones in their blood, even though their glands are healthy. Researchers believe these hormonal irregularities may explain some of the symptoms of depressive illness such as appetite changes, disturbed sleep, and irregular menstrual cycles in women, since hormones are involved in all of these functions.

It has also been shown that people suffering from certain endocrine disorders sometimes experience depression. And, in some people with depression, the endocrine system develops problems even though their glands are healthy. Hormonal irregularities in depressed people may be linked to the fluctuations in brain chemistry found in depressive illness. The brain and the endocrine system are connected at the hypothalamus. The hypothalamus, a small gland in the center of the brain, controls body activities such as appetite, sleep, and sexual desire. It also controls the body's master gland the pituitary gland, which regulates the secretion of hormones from many other glands. In running the endocrine system the hypothalamus uses some of the same neurotransmitters that have been linked to depression; norepinephrine, serotonin, and dopamine [14].

Cortisol, a hormone released by the adrenal gland during times of stress has been observed in high levels by depressed people. High levels of cortisol in the blood stream typically return to normal when the depression lifts. In many depressed people the hypothalamus which controls the release of cortisol appears to be faulty, and does not shut off Researchers have found the more cortisol in the bloodstream, the less of certain mood-altering neurotransmitters are present. This suggests that something controlling cortisol levels, whether the hypothalamus or some other part of the brain, may influence depression [15].

Genetic Causes

Genetics appears to also play a role in the prevalence of depression. Depressive illness is believed to be partly hereditary because research on families shows that some are more prone to developing depression than others. Studies on twins has shown whether identical twins grew up together or apart the prevalence of the other twin having depressive illness when the other did was 67 percent greater than not. Whereas, fraternal twins showed a prevalence rate of only 19 percent of the time. Scientists first identified a gene linked to depressive illness in 1987. This gene, found on chromosome 11, was reported to carry the susceptibility to bipolar depression. Additional research has pointed to a gene on the X chromosome may also play a role in bipolar depression.

Other studies of families prone to bipolar depression have reported that genes on chromosomes 6, 13, and 15 may also influence the illness. Studies of families prone to manic depression also found a statistical link between the illness and a variation on chromosome 4. Researchers also found a connection between a gene on chromosome 18 and a predisposition to manic depression. Genes on the same part of this chromosome have also been found to affect a protein that allows neurons to receive messages from neurotransmitters. Another gene on chromosome 18 controls some of the body's stress hormones, which are often disturbed in depressive illness [16].

Today, it appears that scientists believe that no one gene, but a number of genes may make someone susceptible to depressive illness. No research so far has drawn a definite link between a specific gene and a predisposition to depressive illness in all people. Some gene, however, may carry a predisposition in certain families. Some scientists believe that many genes act together to make someone susceptible. It is estimated that if you inherit a gene that makes you susceptible you have between a 50 and 70 percent chance of developing a depressive disorder. This means that an individual has a one-third or more chance of getting a depressive illness that is controlled by environmental factors [17].

Environmental Causes

Environmental factors that may lead to a depressive illness include stressful or traumatic events. Events such as a loss of a spouse or close relative, loss of a job, or end of a relationship may lead to depression. Many people with depressive illness can point to a traumatic event that preceded their illness. However, many people struggle with hurtful changes at some time in their lives and do not develop depressive illness. And, some people develop depressive illness when everything in their life is going well. Many researchers believe environmental influences act in combination with genetic predisposition to depressive illness to foster depression [18].

Researchers believe a loss or crisis is more likely to precede a first or second episode of depression. After those initial episodes, however, subsequent episodes often occur spontaneously. It is unclear why stressful life events are more likely to precede the first episodes of depression than the later episodes. But, according to one theory, the first episode may lead to long-lasting changes in the chemistry of the brain. This theory, called the kindling-sensitization hypothesis, suggests that the initial episode kindles, or sparks, long-lasting (or permanent) changes in the brain's limbic system, making it more sensitive to future episodes. Because the first episode increases a person's vulnerability to depression, minor stressful events can more easily set off later episodes [19].

Depression has been associated with stressful situations such as low self-esteem, high self criticism, significant cognitive distortions, and a feeling of lack of control over negative events. The cognitive-diathesis model proposes that individuals who are exposed to stressful events and who have negative styles of interpreting and coping with stress are at high risk of developing depressive symptoms. Studies have suggested that certain behaviors such as criticism, rejection, and experiences with uncontrollable stressful life events, may play a role in depression. Depressed children and adolescents have been shown to have increased cognitive distortions, negative attributions, hopelessness, tendency to attribute outcomes to external non-controllable causes, social skill deficits, and low self-esteem compared with non-affective psychiatric and normal controls [20].

Physical Causes

Depression can have several physical causes beyond the neurotransmitter or hormonal imbalances previously discussed. **Thyroid disease**, extremely common especially among women, is often accompanied by depression. In some cases depression and fatigue may be the first signs of thyroid disease. Both kinds of thyroid disease, hypothyroidism, where the thyroid secretes too little hormone, and hyperthyroidism, where too much hormone is secreted can cause depression. But depression is more likely to accompany hypothyroidism.

Diseases of the adrenal gland can also cause depression. **Addison's disease** in which the adrenal cortex gradually stops functioning can promote depression. In **Cushing's syndrome,** the level of corticosteroid hormone in the blood is too high due to an overactive adrenal gland, which can also lead to depression.

Hyperparathyroidism, a condition in which the parathyroid gland produces too much parathyroid hormone can give rise to depression. This hormone increases the amount of calcium in the blood a condition called hypercalcemia, and can cause excessive urination, tiredness, nausea, and vomiting [21].

Complications from **diabetes mellitus** can cause depression. Diabetes is a disease where the pancreas produces little or insulin, the hormone that regulates glucose in the blood stream. Physical complications from diabetes include eye, nerve, kidney, and circulation problems, which in turn can make a person depressed. As many as one fourth of all people with diabetes mellitus also develop depressive illness [22].

Infectious diseases such as **mononucleosis, hepatitis** or **pneumonia** can give rise to depression, as a symptom of the disease or as a psychological response to the illness. Depression is often an early sign of mononucleosis, a viral disease that causes flu-like symptoms, headache, and weakness. If depression does not develop early in the illness, it may do so near the end of the illness and be the last symptom to clear up.

In **viral hepatitis** (type A, B, or C) depression is common at any stage of the disease. **Viral pneumonia** is an inflammation of the lungs caused by a virus. Depression or mental confusion often accompanies this illness. **Chronic Fatigue Syndrome** (CFS), an illness many researchers believe is caused by viruses. Symptoms of CFS include flu-like symptoms, total exhaustion, joint and muscle weakness and pain, swollen glands, sore throat, headaches, forgetfulness, and confusion. CFS primarily occurs in women between the ages of 25 and 45, and can strike suddenly and last for months or years. Because depression usually always accompanies CFS, some researchers believe it may be a form of depressive illness [23].

Many people who have cancer develop major depression as a psychological response to the disease. However, some tumors can secrete serotonin, causing an imbalance that produces symptoms of depression. Brain tumors are among the cancers most likely to give rise to depression, and may be the earliest or only symptom of the tumor [24].

Autoimmune disorders, diseases of the immune system, such as **lupus** or **HIV/AIDS** have been linked to depression. Systemic lupus erythematosus (SLE), which causes the body's connective tissue to become inflamed, damaging the skin, joints, and internal organs, can bring about mental changes as well, including depression. Depression occurs in about 10 percent of people who are infected with the human immunodeficiency virus (HIV), the virus that gives rise to the acquired immunodeficiency syndrome (AIDS). When the HIV develops into AIDS depression develops in at least 30 percent of cases [25].

Degenerative disorders can cause depression. Between one third and one half of the people that develop Parkinson's disease, which causes progressive deterioration of the nervous system, develop depression. **Huntington's chorea** a hereditary, degenerative nerve disease causes uncontrollable body movements and mental deterioration. Depression, euphoria, or other mental changes sometimes mark the early stages of Huntington's chorea.

Multiple sclerosis, another degenerative disease of the nervous system, may show symptoms of mood changes and depression, often years before the illness is diagnosed. Depression is seen in up to 87 percent of the cases reported in people with dementia diseases such as **Alzheimer's Disease**. Dementia and Alzheimer's are characterized by progressive loss of memory and other intellectual functions and is accompanied by depression, paranoia or delusions [26].

Diseases of the cardiovascular system such as heart disease and stroke can cause depression. Among people who experience a heart attack, 15 to 20 percent will develop clinical depression afterward. **Stroke,** which occurs when a rupture or blockage of a blood vessel causes injury to the brain, is a significant cause of depression. Stoke leads to depression in about half of all people hospitalized with the illness. Symptoms of depression in stroke patients may be a result of changes in or damage to the brain caused by the stroke, or a reaction to the physical side effects and limitations caused by the stroke such as paralysis [27].

Diseases of metabolism, the process by which the body converts food and oxygen into energy, may lead to symptoms of depression. Acute intermittent porphyia is one group of very rare diseases caused by an inherited defect in the enzymes that produce a constituent of blood. The disease attacks the nervous system, and symptoms can include nausea, vomiting, constipation, muscle weakness, vision problems, paralysis, and mental changes. Depression is common in acute intermittent porphyria, especially between attacks [28].

Nutritional Deficiencies

Essential nutrient deficiencies may also lead to depression. Prolonged vitamin deficiencies can bring on depression. Depression is a symptom of the disease pellagra, a disease caused by lack of niacin and B-complex vitamins in the diet. Depression and other mental changes can also be early signs that the body lacks vitamin B_{12}. If untreated, vitamin B_{12} deficiency leads to pernicious anemia, which can cause a severe depletion of red blood cells in the body.

Depression can also be a sign that your body is lacking folic acid, vitamin B_6 (pyridoxine), or vitamin B_1 (thiamin). Depression may be the result of a lack of certain essential minerals. Anemia may be the result of an iron deficiency. Depression may also be the result of a shortage in the body's supply of sodium, magnesium, or zinc [29, 30].

Researchers reporting in the May, 2008 issue of *Archives of General Psychiatry* have linked low blood levels of vitamin D and increased parathyroid hormone levels to depression among older adults. They believe when the body lacks the proper amount of vitamin D, the parathyroid produces too much parathyroid hormone. Overactive parathyroid glands, or hyperparathyroidism, often accompany symptoms of depression. In a study of 1,282 adults aged 65 to 95 with depression symptoms, more than a third of the men and over half of the woman were found to be deficient in vitamin D. They also were found to have higher levels of the parathyroid hormone [31].

Dr. Carl Pfeiffer, who founded the **Brain Bio Center** in New Jersey believed that nutrient deficiencies cause mental illness. By testing the blood chemistry of thousands of patients at the center since 1966, Dr. Pfeiffer had determined that the histamine levels are related to mental illness. Histamine is a brain chemical that regulates reactions such as pain and allergies. In a study involving thousands of schizophrenic patients it was found that over 50 percent have low levels of histamine in their blood which is called histapenia. However, high levels of histamine in the blood, a condition called histadelia, is linked to hyperactivity, compulsive behavior, and depression. Unlike low histimine, high levels in the blood appears to be mostly an inherited trait. Histadelics also have symptoms of increased mucus and saliva, have allergies, and periodic headaches [32].

Medication Causes

Prescription medication can cause depression. Research has shown that more than 200 medications have caused depression in certain individuals, but doctors known of only a few that frequently cause depression. Medications for high blood pressure such as reserpine, methyldopa, guanethine, propranolol, and clonidine, can cause significant depression in some people. Drugs used to treat Parkinson's disease such as l-dopa can cause depression and mild mania.

Nonsteroidal anti-inflammatory drugs (NSAIDs) used to relieve pain in osteoarthritis, rheumatoid arthritis, and other joint diseases can cause depression. Anticonvulsant medications used to treat seizure disorders like phenobarbital is particularly likely to bring on depression. Corticosteroid medications used to treat Addison's disease, allergies, rheumatic disorders, and inflammation can cause mental changes including depression in about 5 percent of the people that use these medications. Oral contraceptives are believed to cause depression in women who are susceptible to depression [33].

Allopathic Treatment:

The most common treatments for depressive illness are medication, psychotherapy or a combination of the two. Medications are used to treat depression and mania, especially severe major depression and bipolar depression. Major depression is usually treated with an antidepressant. Antidepressants work by altering the brain's supply of neurotransmitters, the chemical messages used by the brain to send messages and regulate emotions.

Antidepressants:

Antidepressants are divided into categories based on the effect they have on brain chemistry. Studies have shown that a combination of pharmacotherapy and psychotherapy works better than either treatment alone. However, clinical trials of psychotropic medications have shown that placebos used in the trails to be 50 percent as effective as the medication. And, typically 20 to 35 percent of patients fail to respond at all to antidepressant medication. All antidepressant medications have incidence of side effects that may range from mild (such as dry mouth, nausea, headaches) to severe (internal bleeding, coma, death) [34, 35].

Tricyclic Antidepressants

Tricyclic antidepressants are a group of medications that have been used the longest to treat depression. They get their name from their chemical structure that is composed of three rings. Imipramine, one of the first tricyclics, was first developed for schizophrenia. However, it was found to do little to control schizophrenia, but it did lift people's moods. Imipramine is still prescribed today under the brand names *Norfranil, Presamine,* and *Tofranil.* Other tricyclics include amitriptyine, *Endep, Elavil, Amitid*, amoxapine, clomipramine, desipramine, doxepin, maprotiline, nortriptyline, and protriptyline. They work by blocking the reuptake of norepinephrine, a mood-altering neurotransmitter, thereby increasing the amount of norepinephrine in the brain. Some may also block the reuptake of serotonin. Tricyclic antidepressants block reuptake almost immediately, but it usually takes several weeks to take effect [36].

Tricyclic antidepressants also effect other neurotransmitters that help regulate certain body processes. This leads to side effects such as sleepiness, drowsiness, dry mouth, constipation, difficulty urinating, vision problems, dizziness, or a racing heart. Less common side effects are rashes, sweating, tremors, delayed or reduced sexual functioning, weight gain, and dry eyes [37, 38].

Monoamine Oxidase Inhibitors

Monoamine oxidase inhibitors (MAOIs) have been used since the 1950s to treat depression. MAIOs work by preventing monamine oxidase, a substance found in nerve endings, from doing its job. Monamine oxidase breaks down the neurotransmitters norepinephrine, dopamine, and serotonin. When a MAOI is taken fewer of these neurotransmitters are broken down, leaving the brain with a larger supply and an improved mood. Like tricyclics, MAOIs take a few weeks to show any improvement in lifting depression. Side effects include dizziness, changes in blood pressure, weight gain, sleepiness or insomnia, reduced sexual functioning, swollen ankles and fingers. Less frequent side effect can be dry mouth, constipation, blurred vision, and difficulty urinating [39, 40].

Monoamine oxidase also plays a role in breaking down tyramine, a substance found naturally in certain foods. Tyramine raises blood pressure, however, if a MAIO is taken it prevents monoamine oxidase from controlling tyramine. Tyramine can flood the bloodstream, raise blood pressure significantly, and cause throbbing headaches, nausea, vomiting, stroke, heart attack and even death. Therefore, anyone on a MAIO must avoid consuming foods containing tyramine. The list of foods to be avoided includes: chocolate, cheese, sour cream, fermented sausage such as pepperoni, and salami, pastrami and corned beef, tofu, soy sauce, teriyaki, salted, pickled or smoked fish, caviar and escargot, sauerkraut and pickles, fava beans, lima beans, Italian beans, pea pods, yeast products, avocados and dried figs. In addition, alcohol including nonalcoholic beer, caffeinated coffee, tea, and soft drinks should be avoided [41].

Selective Serotonin Reuptake Inhibitors

Selective serotonin reuptake inhibitors (SSRIs) are newer medications used for depression. SSRIs include fluoxetine *(Prozac)*, paroxetine *(Paxil)*, fluvoxamine *(Luvox)*, and sertraline *(Zoloft)*. SSRIs work by increasing the brain's supply of serotonin by blocking the reuptake at the synapse. Because SSRIs target only serotonin they tend to produce fewer side effects than tricyclics or MAIOs. Side effects can include insomnia, nervousness, agitation, nausea, diarrhea, and headaches. Occasionally SSRIs can cause sexual side effects such as diminished interest in sex, arousal problems, and difficulty achieving organism [42, 43, 44].

Atypical Antidepressants

Atypical antidepressants include bupropion *(Wellbutrin)*, trazodone *(Desyrel)*, venlafaxine hydrochloride *(Effexor)*, nefazodone hydrochloride *(Serzone)*, and mirtazapine *(Remeron)*. Bupropion is believed to work by blocking the reuptake of dopamine. It is less likely than other antidepressants to cause weight gain and sexual problems. Its side effects may include excitement, agitation, sleeplessness, nausea and tremor. Bupropion may also cause seizures in high doses. Trazodone works by blocking the reuptake of serotonin. It may also have side effects of digestive problems, bad breath, nausea, or a rapid heartbeat. It may make blood pressure drop slightly and can cause abnormal heart rhythms. Venlafaxine hydrochloride also blocks the reuptake of serotonin. Possible side effects include sleeplessness, dizziness and headaches. A new FDA warning (10/08) reports a higher risk of fatal overdoses when *Effexor* is taken with alcohol or other SSRIs. Nefazodone hydrochloride increases the amount of serotonin and norepinephrine in the brain. Its possible side effects include sleeplessness, increased blood pressure and blurred vision. Mirtazapine works by stimulating the release of serotonin and norepinephrine and is less likely to cause sexual problems, but may cause drowsiness, increased appetite, weight gain, and dizziness [45, 46, 47, 48].

Lithium

Lithium carbonate (*Eskalith*) is used to treat both depression and the mania of bipolar disease. Lithium was first developed in the 1940's as a salt substitute for people on low sodium diets. However, early doses of lithium salts were too high and people were poisoned and some even died. In 1949 an Australian researcher discovered guinea pigs treated with lithium remained calm. By the 1960's lithium was used in several countries to treat bipolar illness and approved for use in the U.S. in 1974.

Lithium may work by slowing down the chemical reactions in neurons or they may block certain proteins that help regulate certain neurotransmitters, researchers are not quite certain. About 40 percent of people on lithium experience side effects of digestive problems like nausea, vomiting, diarrhea, and stomachaches. Excessive urination, tremors, weight gain, acne, dry skin, headaches, sleeplessness and exhaustion are also often experienced. Lithium will interact with medications such as aspirin, ibuprofen and the antibiotic tetracycline, increasing the levels of lithium in the blood to dangerous levels [49, 50].

Anticonvulsants

Several medications developed to treat seizures also help bipolar depression. These drugs called anticonvulsants include valproic acid, divalproex sodium, and clonazepam. In doing so, it calms nerves that control muscle movement and prevents seizures. In high doses carbamazepine can damage the liver and interfere with the production of blood cells in the bone marrow. Typical side effects include dizziness, drowsiness, headaches, double vision, nausea, diarrhea, and skin rash. Valproic acid and divalproex sodium are prescribed if lithium or carbamazepine are not effective in preventing mood swings. They also have similar side effects of stomach disorders, drowsiness and can make hair fall out. Clonazepam does not even out an individual's mood, but it does relieve some of mania's effects. It is often prescribed with lithium. Side effects of clonazepam includes sleeplessness, clumsiness, and psychotic experiences. Carbamazepine, an antiepileptic, works by blocking an amino acid called gamma-aminobutyric acid (GABA), and has a host of similar side-effects (see table 5-1) [51, 52, 53].

Antipsychotics

A newly FDA approved medication Areipiprazole (*Abilify*) has also been approved for the treatment of depression when it is used with antidepressants.

Abilify is classified as an antipsychotic drug used in the treatment of schizophrenia and bipolar disorder. It is believed to work by modifying the sensitivity of serotonin and dopamine. Common side effects could include abnormal dreams, anxiety, blurred vision, chest pain, constipation, flu-like symptoms, headache, insomnia, rash and weight gain. The risk of tardive dyskinesia, as in permanent facial tics, increases with the total amount of *Abilify* taken. In rare cases *Abilify* has been known to cause a potentially fatal condition known as Neuroleptic Malignant Syndrome (NMS). Symptoms include high fever, rigid muscles, irregular pulse and blood pressure, rapid heartbeat excessive perspiration, and altered mental status [54].

TMS & ECT

The FDA approved a **transcranial magnetic stimulation** (TMS) device for use in treating depression in adults that antidepressant medication has failed to work on. The TMS uses a magnetic field to induce a small electric current in a specific part of the brain. In clinical trials it was shown to benefit patients with mild depression. Patients are treated 4 to 5 times a week with a TMS device in a doctor's office. Neuronetics Inc. are the makers of the TMS device NeuroStar that was approved for use by the FDA [55].

TMS therapy is reported to be much safer than **electroconvulsive therapy** (ECT). ECT also known as electroshock therapy, that uses an electric shock to induce a seizure and is recommended for severely depressed patients that do not respond to medication. An ECT patient has to be sedated during treatment and is usually conducted on patients that are hospitalized [56].

Table 5-1
Summary of Allopathic Treatment for Depression [35, 36, 37:]

Drug: *(Brand name)*	Acting mechanism:	Possible side effects:
Tricyclic Antidepressants: **Amitid, Amoxapine** *(Asendin),* **Amitriptyine** *(Elavil, Endep, Etrafon, Levate, Novo- Doxepin, Novotriptyn, PMS-Amitriptyline, Triavil).* **Clomipramine** *(Anafranil)* **Desipramine** *(Norpranmin)* **Doxepin** *(Adapin Novo-Doxepin, Sinequan)* **Imipramine** *(Norfranil, Presamine, Tofranil)* **Nortriptyline** *(Aventyl, Pamelor),* **Trimipramine maleate** *(Surmontil)* **Protriptyline** *(PMS-Levazine, Triptil,* Vivactil,*	Blocks the reuptake of norepinephrine, a mood-altering neurotransmitter. Some may also block the reuptake of serotonin.	**Common:** Tremors, headache, dry mouth, constipation or diarrhea, nausea, indigestion, fatigue, weakness, drowsiness, nervousness, anxiety, excessive sweating, insomnia, weight gain, dry eyes. **Infrequent:** convulsions, hallucinations, dizziness, fainting, blurred vision, vomiting, irregular heartbeat, inflamed tongue, abdominal pain, jaundice, hair loss, rash, fever, chills, joint pain, palpitations, urination difficulty, decreased sex drive, muscle aches, abnormal dreams, nasal congestion, back pain.

Monoamine Oxidase Inhibitors (MAOIs): **Moclobemide** *(Man*erix*)*, **Phenelzine** *(Nardil, Hydrazine)*, **Selegiling** *(Eldepryl)*, **Tranylcypromine** *(Parnate, Nonhydrazine)*	Blocks monoamine oxidase an enzyme involved in the metabolic decomposition and inactivation of norepinephrine, Serotonin and dopamine.	Decreased heart rate, decreased vasoconstriction, hypotension, dry mouth, blurred vision, constipation, urinary hesitation, agitation, anxiety, restlessness, insomnia, euphoria, hypomania. MAOI's react negatively with other anti-depressants, anticholinergic drugs, anesthetics, antihypertensives, amphetamines and tyramine-rich foods (alcoholic beverages, cheese, sour cream, yogurt, processed meats, caffeine, chocolate, licorice, soy sauce and yeast).
Selective Serotonin Reuptake Inhibitors (SSRI's): **Citalopram** *(Celexa)*, **Duloxetine hydrochloride** *(Cymbalta)*, **Escitalopram** *(Lexapro)*, **Fluoxetine** *(Prozac, Sarafem, Symbyax)*, **Fluvoxamine** *(Luvox)*, **Paroxetine** *(Paxil)*, **Sertraline** *(Zoloft)*	Blocks the reuptake of serotonin, a neuro-transmitter.	Drowsiness, nausea, back pain, mouth/lip sores, constipation or diarrhea, headache, anxiety, sexual side-effects, insomnia, dry mouth. **Infrequent:** vision changes, confusion, apathy, breathing difficulty, chills, fever, enlarged lymph glands, irregular heartbeat, vomiting, skin rash, appetite loss, urinary changes, muscle or joint pain, menstrual changes, loss of hair, seizures.

Atypical Antidepressants: **Bupropion** *(Wellbutrin)* **Mirtazapine** *(Remeron)*, **Nefazodone** *(Serazone)* **Trazodone** *(Desyrel)* **Venlafaxine** *(Effexor, Pristiq)*	Inhibits serotonin, norepinephrine, dopamine reuptake. Blocks specific (5HT) neurotransmitters.	Nausea, dry mouth, dizziness, constipation, nervousness, sweating, anorexia, hyper-tension, agitation, insomnia, gastro-intestinal upset, headache.
Antiepileptic: **Carbamazepine** *(Carbatrol, Mazepine, Tegretol)*	Normalizes sodium channel activity and sodium influx, dopamine and nor-epinephrine.	CNS drowsiness, dizziness, confusion, fatigue, paralysis, headache, hallucinations, nausea, vomiting, fever, hypertension or hypotension, chills, rash, blood dyscrasias (aplastic anemia, leucopoenia, aganulocytosis, thrombocytopenia, bone marrow depression).

Effectiveness of Antidepressants

A study conducted by a former FDA researcher found that many antidepressant studies exaggerate their effectiveness. In the study, 12 commonly prescribed antidepressants that were approved by the FDA between 1987 and 2004 were scrutinized. The study looked at 74 FDA registered studies, involving 12,564 patients, comparing FDA reviews of the studies with study reviews published in medical journals. They found that the published results didn't always jibe with the FDA review of the study. They found that of the 36 studies that had negative or questionable results, 22 were not published in medical journals, and 11 were published in way that appeared to be positive (when they had negative results). While the FDA concluded that 51% of these studies had positive results for the antidepressants, the published literature reported that 94% of the studies had positive results [57].

Naturopathic Treatment

Alternative medicine, which the medical community now describes as complimentary medicine includes theories and practices such as herbal medicine, homeopathy, therapeutic touch, and imagery. Alternative remedies have found their way into the medical mainstream today. Medical schools teach alternative medicine, hospitals and health maintenance organizations offer it and laws in some states require plans to cover it. It also constitutes a huge and rapidly growing industry in which major pharmaceutical companies are now participating in [58].

The National Institutes of Health, in Bethesda, MD, estimate that only 10 to 30 percent of the health care worldwide is allopathic, or "western". The rest of the world's medical care is what Americans would call alternative. Western medicine often appears to be quick to criticize alternative treatments, however, the *Harvard Mental Health Letter* (2/05) reports that in recent clinical trials of antidepressants it was reported that there was little or no difference in the therapeutic effect between the drug and a placebo [59].

St. John's wort

The medical community's most significant concern over complimentary medicine appears to be the lack of clinical studies that verify claims made for them. However, a substantial body of evidence is now available for the effectiveness of **St. John's wort** *Hypericum perforatum*, in treating depression.

St. John's wort is believed to have been used for more than 2,000 years for nervous disorders. It grows as a common weed through much of the United States and its yellow flower was traditionally gathered for the feast of St. John the Baptist and harvested on June 24th. Wort is the Old English word for plant or herb, hence the derivation of its common name [60].

From the time of the ancient Greeks through the Middle Ages, St. John's wort was considered magical and used to ward off evil and protect against disease, heal wounds, remedy kidney troubles, alleviate nervous disorders, and even cure insanity [61]. Reports of St. John's wort use date back to the first century Greek botanist Dioscorides, first century Roman scholar, Pliny and fifth century Greek physician, Hippocrates. Uses of the herb ranged in curing such illnesses as anxiety, colds, depression, flu, hemorrhoids, menstrual cramps, skin infections, cuts and burns [62]. As scientific studies developed in the nineteenth century research supported the use of St. John's wort for mood disorders. The first study on St. John's wort was published in 1939.

St. John's wort's popularity as a treatment for depression grew throughout

Europe, and it was officially approved as antidepressant drug in 1988 in Germany. By 1993 Germany physicians issued more than 2.7 million prescriptions for St. John's wort. Currently German physicians prescribe St. John's wort 8 times more often than Prozac. Interest in the herb has gradually increased in the U.S. to where sales for St. John's wort grew from $20 million in 1990 to $200 million in 1997 [63].

Early research on St. John's wort believed it worked by inhibiting the enzyme monoamine-oxidase. However, these studies involved applying extracts of St. John's wort directly into test tubes and later investigation showed that the dosages taken orally are 100 times too low to inhibit monamine-oxidase. More recent research suggests that St. John's wort may function more like the SSRIs by inhibiting the reuptake of serotonin. In laboratory studies, hyperforin, an ingredient in St. John's wort inhibits the reuptake of serotonin, dopamine, and norepinephrine [64].

According to the National Institute of Mental Health, St. John's wort may modulate the activity of interleukin-6 (Il-6), a protein involved in the communication between cells in the body's immune system. Il-6 may lead to increases in adrenal regulatory hormones a suspected cause of depression. St John's wort may reduce levels of Il-6, thus helping to ease depression [65].

In a meta-analysis study by Linde et al (1996), 23 randomized controlled trials involving 1,757 outpatients suffering from mild to moderate depression were reviewed. Fifteen of the trials were placebo controlled, and 8 compared St. John's wort to antidepressants. The overall responder rate showed that St. John's wort was significantly superior to placebo, and was found to have an efficacy similar to that of standard antidepressants. Compared with the antidepressant groups, St. John's wort had lower dropout rates (7.7 % to 4 %) and numbers of patients reporting adverse effects (35.9 % to 19.8 %). 81 percent of the participants taking St. John's wort improved significantly, while only 26 percent of the placebo group improved. Comparative analysis of adverse effects concluded that St. John's wort seems to be at least as safe and possibly safer than conventional antidepressant drugs and is highly effective for treating mild to moderate depression [66].

In a comparable study in 2008 reviewing 29 trials of St. John's wort involving 5,489 people similar results were reported. The reviewers concluded that St. John's wort was more effective than placebo and had fewer side effects than similar antidepressants. The study also reported that St. John's wort is commonly prescribed in Germany for depression, anxiety and sleep disorders [67].

Typical dosages of St. John's wort in order to achieve therapeutic benefit is 300 mg, three times a day of a standardized extract of 0.3 percent hypericin. Higher doses are not believed to produce greater benefits, and like prescription antidepressants, St. John's wort typically takes 4 to 6 weeks to be effective. Due to occasional stomach irritation it should be taken with food.

Side-effect incidence of St. John's wort is extremely minimal when comparing it to prescription antidepressants (35.9 %). In a study involving 3,250 patients taking St. John's wort extract for 4 weeks, the most common side effect was mild stomach discomfort reported in 0.6 percent of the patients. Allergic reactions such as skin rashes and itching developed in 0.5 percent, tiredness in 0.4 percent, and restlessness in 0.3 percent. The total percentage of patients reporting side effects in the study was 2.4 percent. In another study, 7.4 percent of patients taking St. John's wort reported an adverse effect compared with 6.2 percent taking a placebo.

In four trials comparing St. John's wort with patients taking prescription antidepressants, those taking the antidepressants were 33 to 78 percent more likely to experience adverse effects than those taking St. John's wort [68, 69]. Fewer than 1 percent of patients in the clinical trials dropped out because of the side effects from St. John's wort, compared to 3 percent of standard prescription medications [70]. Although none of the patients in these studies experienced photosensitivity, it has been listed as a possible side effect. In a study by Brockmoller [71], twice the recommended dosage of St. John's wort (1,800 mg per day) was given to 50 healthy volunteers and at the end of 15 days the time required to cause a sunburn increased by 21 percent. Therefore, people who are photosensitive (light skinned) should monitor their intake of St. John's wort and their time in the sun when not wearing a sunscreen.

The frequency and severity of side effects with St. John's wort are clinically insignificant, especially when compared to the well-known side effects of tricyclics and other antidepressants. There have been no deaths due to St. John's wort toxicity, a stark contrast to the 31 deaths per one million prescriptions produced by the synthetic antidepressants [72].

The FDA has warned about possible drug interactions when using St. John's wort. The warning was based on a study conducted by the National Institute of Health where healthy patients received indinavir, a protease inhibitor used in HIV infection treatment and 900 mg per day of St. John's wort. In the study, St. John's wort decreased the effectiveness of indinavir plasma concentration.

Another report suggests the herb causes similar drops in plasma levels of cyclosporine after heart transplants. It is believed St. John's wort may have a similar effect on nonnucleoside reverse transcriptase inhibitors (NNRTIs) such as delavirdine, efavirenz, and nevirapine that utilize the same metabolic pathway as the herb. Other medications that use this pathway that St. John's wort may reduce their effectiveness may include: antidepressants like imipramine, amoxapine, or amitriptyline, heart medications such as digoxin, diltiazem, nifedipine, digitoxin, x-beta-blockers, seizure medications like carbamazepine, phenytoin, or phenobarbital, cancer treatment medications such as cyclophosphamide, tamoxifen, taxol, or etoposide, transplant rejection drugs such as cyclosporine, rapamycin or tacrolimus and ethinyl estradiol for pregnancy [73, 74].

The positive side effects of appear to greatly out number the negative side effects reported in St. John's wort use. In addition to reducing depression St. John's wort has been observed to improve mood, decrease anxiety, increase self-esteem, improve sleep, improve concentration, relieve seasonal affective disorder, reduce headache frequency, reduce gastrointestinal symptoms, improve exhaustion symptoms and reduce leg muscle pain [75, 76].

Research conducted in Russia on St. John's wort found it effective in treating alcoholics suffering from depression when combined with psychotherapy. A major advantage of St. John's wort found in this study was that unlike antidepressant drugs it does not impair attention, concentration or reaction time [77]. St. John's wort has been found to be as effective in treating mild to moderate depression, just as Prozac is reported to be. Dr. Peter Kramer, *Listening To Prozac,* states that Prozac may be effective in treating minor depression, not major depressive illness as originally thought [78].

SAMe

S-Adenosylmethionine (SAMe) was first discovered in 1953 in Italy. It became a popular remedy for depression and commercially produced in for depression in Europe in 1977. It was not available in the U.S. until 1999. SAMe is formed in the body by a combination of ATP and the amino acid, methionine. It plays a key role in numerous metabolic pathways involving the transfer of methyl groups.

SAMe is believed to work by either increasing the synthesis of neurotransmitters such as serotonin and norepinephrine and increasing the responsiveness of neurotransmitter receptors or it increases the fluidity of cell membranes of phospholipids. The most significant adverse effect of SAMe is mania, manifested by pressured speech and a display of grandiose ideas, others have reported nausea [79].

In clinical studies comparing SAMe and tricyclics, SAMe out-performed the tricyclics in treating depression. The tricyclics used in the study were amitriptyline, chlorimipramine, imipramine and desipramine, all in therapeutic doses. The dosages for SAMe were 200 to 400 mg intravenously or 1,600 mg orally per day. The response rate for SAMe was 61 percent and for the tricyclics 59 percent.

Another study measured the response rate (how quickly effects are noticed) of SAMe for depression. In the study, 195 patients were given 400 mg intramuscularly (IM) of SAMe daily and showed a response rate of 7 to 14 days. This compares to a minimum of 21 days for other antidepressants.

A study compared the onset of response to a combination of SAMe (200 mg, IM/day) with an antidepressant, imipramine (150 mg orally/day) versus imipramine alone. Results of the study indicated depressive illness symptoms decreased more rapidly with the combination of imipramine and SAMe, than with imipramine alone. The study also indicated SAMe can be combined with antidepressants resulting in positive effects and in doing so the dose of the antidepressant can be reduced, reducing the side effects of the antidepressant. SAMe appears to be as effective orally as it is when administered intramuscularly or intravenously. For antidepressant treatment 1,600 mg per day (2 doses of 800 mg, or 4 of 400 mg) is recommended [80].

Ginkgo

A number of studies from Germany supports the use of ginkgo *(Ginkgo biloba)* as an antidepressant. Ginkgo, a tree that is indigenous to China has been used to treat a number of illnesses in China for close to 5,000 years. Chinese healers have used it to treat such wide-ranging ills as asthma, bladder infections, chronic coughing, headaches, memory problems, premature ejaculation, and tuberculosis. Ginkgo trees are deciduous trees that can grow to 120 feet, and live for nearly 4,000 years. It has leathery, fan-shaped leaves that turn gold in autumn with smelly apricot-sized fruits that contain large seeds or nuts. Although the leaves are also utilized in Asia, the seeds and seed oil are more commonly used, whereas, in North America and Europe the leaves are usually used medicinally [81].

Researchers have isolated certain active ingredients they believe are responsible for the healing properties of ginkgo. Ginkgo has two main types of active ingredients, flavone glycosides and terpene lactones. Flavone glycosides are a type of flavonoids or antioxidants, found in a number of plants and fruits. In addition to working as antioxidants, these compounds strengthen the capillary walls, reduce inflammation, and help prevent bruising. Specific flavone glycosides in ginkgo include quercetin, kaempferol, and isorhamnetin. The optimal level of flavone glycoside in ginkgo is 22 to 27 percent of the active ingredients in the product. Terpene lactones are unique to the ginkgo tree and include bilobalides and ginkgolides. These compounds help thin the blood, prevent blood clots, improve circulation to the brain, help the body use glucose more effectively and protects from nerve damage during oxygen deprivation. Researchers believe ginkgo's effect in alleviating depression has to do with its ability to increase the supply of oxygen to the brain [82].

The Germany Ministry of Health Committee for Herbal Remedies approves ginkgo as a treatment for depression, improving mood and mental processes. In a study they conducted of individuals between the ages of 51 to 78 that did not respond to antidepressant medication marked improvement was recorded after 4 weeks of treatment of 240 mg. per day of ginkgo. They believe the herb helps combat depression by increasing blood flow to the brain making it function more efficiently, and by increasing brain levels of dopamine. Although side effects are rare with ginkgo use some users have reported minor side effects of dizziness, upset stomach (4 percent of users), and mild headache (very rare) [83].

Ginseng

Ginseng, *Panax ginseng,* is a herb that has been used for centuries to boost energy, sharpen the mind, reduce stress, reverse impotence, enhance the immune system, control blood pressure, regulate blood-sugar, and strengthen the cardiovascular system. In traditional Chinese medicine ginseng is considered a superior medicine because it is credited with restoring or balancing *qi* or vital life energy. It is believed to balance, harmonize, and strengthen the body's various systems, it helps the body heal itself.

Ginseng's effect in relieving depression is related to its ability to reduce stress. Ginseng improves blood flow to the brain, improving concentration and mental performance. Ginseng may perform its balancing act on the body's systems by strengthening the adrenal glands. It seems to play a role in the regulation of the levels of the hormone ACTH (adrenocorticotropic hormone) in the blood, which in turn stimulates adrenal activity. Ginseng also appears to help the hypothalamus be more effective at controlling stress. The hypothalamus is a gland that plays an important role in regulating hormones that control stress such as corticosterone [84]. Ginseng may also work by operating like an antidepressant, as it is believed to increase the availability of serotonin in the brain [85].

The American Medical Association warns that a potential side effects of ginseng include insomnia, hypertension, diarrhea and anxiety. And, recommend that ginseng should not be taken by patients on hypertension or diabetic medication [86].

Kava kava

Kava kava, *Piper methysticum*, is a herb that has been reportedly used as a treatment for depression, anxiety and sleep aid for some 3,000 years in the South Pacific. St. John's wort is the world's most prescribed herbal antidepressant, but kava ranks just below it. The kava plant is a hardy, flowering shrub belonging to the pepper family. The plant, which reaches maturity in 3 to 5 years has heart-shaped leaves and can grow to 10 feet tall.

Active ingredients of kava are kavalactones which include demthyoxyangonin, dilhydrokavain, yangonin, kavain, dihydromethysticin, and methysticin. Most of these medicinal constituents are found in the roots of the kava plant. Researchers believe kava works as an antidepressant by acting as a central nervous system sedative. The kavalactones in kava appear to target the limbic system, the part of the brain that helps regulate moods and controls emotions.

Recommended dosage of kava is 250 mg, 3 times per day. High doses of kava (over 40,000 mg, per day) have been reported to cause blurred vision, shortness of breath, scale-like skin, reddened eyes, blood in urine, and yellowish discoloration of skin and nails when taking it for several months. Kava is not recommended when taking prescription medication for depression or anxiety, while taking alcohol, for patients with Parkinson's disease (can worsen disease symptoms) or women who are pregnant, trying to conceive or nursing [87].

Lavender

Another herb reported to relieve depression is lavender, *Lavandula officinalis*. Lavender is one of the most distinctively aromatic of the healing herbs with a long history of commercial and medical use. It is used in soaps, perfumes, powders, sachets and even moth repellants.

Herbalists prescribe lavender tea or the essential oil of lavender (used externally) to treat emotional as well as physical problems. Internally, it is available in dried flowers, powdered herb, tea capsules or tincture and is used to treat depression, emotional stress, tension, insomnia, headache, muscle aches, indigestion and nausea. Used externally as aromatherapy, lavender's essential oil is used for relaxation, stimulation of the mind, to clarify thinking, and relieve depression [88].

Natural Therapies:

Aromatherapy

Aromatherapy uses pure essential oils to cure a variety illnesses and diseases. The history of aromatherapy dates back many centuries and the Arabic countries are credited with the process of discovering how to distill oils over a thousand years ago. **Essential oils** are highly concentrated substances, for example, the essential oil of rose may take 5,000 roses to produce 5 ml (1 teaspoon).

Essential oils are used externally in soaps, bath oils, massage oils, and perfumes and internally as teas, powders, and capsules. Many essential oils have a profound effect on mood and may relieve depression. Bergamot is an uplifting oil that has a refreshing citrus fragrance, and it gives Earl Grey tea its distinctive aroma. Clary sage is a relaxing, but uplifting, almost euphoric effect that can relieve chronic tension that can lead to depression. Geranium's essential oil actually comes from varieties of scented pelargonium, and has a tonic effect on the adrenal cortex, which helps to regulate stress hormone production. Neroli is the essential oil from the bitter orange blossom and is reported to relax and sooth and it can relieve muscle spasm and the irritability that often goes with a depressed state [89].

Diet

Natural therapy includes **dietary** considerations in order to treat depression. A poor diet and a lack of essential vitamins can cause depression. Specifically a lack of B-vitamins can cause depression. Junk foods high in sugar and devoid of vitamins places stress on the pancreas and depletes B-vitamins and calcium from the body. Caffeine addiction creates thiamin deficiency and weakens the nervous system. Too much meat causes uric acid and other toxins to accumulate in the blood. Alcohol depletes the body of vitamins and minerals and strains the detoxifying organs such as the liver, kidneys and pancreas.

To counteract the effects of a deficient diet that could lead to depression a multi-vitamin is recommended with extra vitamins A, B-complex (thiamin-B_1, pyridoxine-B_5, B_{12}, folic acid, niacin) and C. Multi-minerals are essential for brain health especially calcium, magnesium, selenium and zinc.

A diet high in complex carbohydrates and protein also has a positive effect against depression. Complex carbohydrates such as brown rice, millet, buckwheat, corn meal, whole wheat, and oats contain tryptophan, an amino acid that has a calming effect. Organically grown turkey breast is high in tryptophan also. Protein creates alertness because it contains dopamine and norepinephrine. Fish is high in protein and good sources include salmon, cod, and tuna. Dry beans are also high in protein. Fresh and steamed vegetables are good sources of minerals like calcium and magnesium essential for brain and nervous system functioning [90].

Dr. Marie-Annette Brown in her book *When Your Body Gets The Blues* (2002), suggests taking three steps to overcome depression, increase your exposure to light, exercise and taking a daily antidepressant "cocktail". By taking a daily walk outdoors the individual gets more light (natural vitamin D) and exercise, both helpful in reducing depression. Her daily depression cocktail consists of: B_1 (thiamin) of 50 mg to relieve fatigue and improve memory, B_2 (riboflavin) 50 mg, for the production of neurotransmitters, B_6 (pyridoxine) 50 mg, to stimulate serotonin production, folic acid, 400 mcg, to help relieve depression, vitamin D, 400 IUs, to stimulate production of serotonin, and selenium, 20 mcg to enhance dopamine activity in the brain [91].

Essential Fatty Acids

Studies with **essential fatty acids** (EFA's) have shown to be effective in treating depression. There are two types of EFA's that are extremely important in nutrition omega-6 EFA's or linoleic acid, and omega-3 EFA's called alpha-linolenic acid. Linoleic acid is often referred to as polyunsaturated and includes gamma-linolenic acid found in borage, hemp, and evening primrose oils and arahidonic acid found in animal products. Both play important roles in the body in behavioral disturbances, healthy skin, hair, liver, kidney and gland function. Alpha-linolenic acid is sometimes referred to as superunsaturated oils and include eiosapentaenoic acid and docosahexaenoic acid. Both are found in fish and seafood, and play important roles in the body such as proper growth, vision, motor and cognitive functioning [92].

Evening primrose oil (omega-6 EFA) has been extensively tested in clinical double blind studies for its therapeutic effects on various diseases. It has been shown to be an adjunctive treatment for schizophrenics, who have low levels of prostaglandin E1, one of several prostaglandins made from EFA's. Prostaglandin E1 levels were increased by giving evening primrose oil which resulted in improvement for schizophrenics. Evening primrose oil has also shown to relieve the symptoms of premenstrual syndrome of depression, irritability, bloating and aggressive behavior.

Studies have shown that humans living in polar regions whose diet consisted of fish and marine animals that provided large quantities of EFA's (omega-3) did not get depressed or suicidal during long winters of total darkness. Whereas, Europeans living north of the Arctic Circle or Western diets suffered "winter blues" and had neurotic, psychotic, and suicidal tendencies. EFA's have been found to be essential in proper brain cell function, and when lacking leads to depressed brain function and behavioral depression [93].

In addition to a deficient diet, excess caffeine and nicotine consumption can lead to depression. Consuming large amounts of caffeine per day can lead to a clinical condition called caffeinism that can cause depression, nervousness, heart palpitations, irritability, recurrent headache, and twitching.

Smoking can effect behavior through the actions of carbon monoxide poisoning of the brain, nicotine poisoning and induction of low levels of vitamin C (smoking depletes vitamin C in the body) which contributes to the classical 'neurotic triad' of hypochondriasis, depression and hysteria. Nicotine stimulates adrenal hormone secretion, adrenaline and cortisol. Cortisol inhibits then uptake of tryptophan by the brain, resulting in decreased serotonin activity in the brain. In addition to not smoking, and reducing caffeine consumption, Drs. Murray and Pizzorno recommend supplementation of B-complex (50 times RDA), 3 grams of vitamin C, 400 mg. of folic acid, 500 mg. of magnesium, 6 grams of tryptophan and 400 mg. of D,L-phenylalanine per day in order to relieve depression [94].

Liver Imbalance

According to Traditional Chinese medicine depression is the result of a stagnant liver. A stagnant liver is considered an imbalance and the *qi* (life force) stagnates in the liver and is not properly distributed. Since it is the *qi* that guides the flow of fluids and nourishment in the body when it is stagnate in the liver, swelling of the liver occurs. The principle cause for this condition is eating too much food especially rich, greasy food that makes the liver become swollen and sluggish. To cure a stagnant liver it is recommended to eat less and eliminate or greatly reduce foods high in saturated fats such as lard, animal meats, cream, cheese, eggs, shortening, margarine, refined and rancid oils, nuts and seeds, alcohol, highly refined and processed foods. Foods that are recommended to treat depression include brown rice, cucumber, apples, cabbage, wheat germ, kuzu root, wild blue-green micro algae (*Aphanizomenon flos-aquae)* and apple cider vinegar [95].

When depressed individuals do not respond to traditional antidepressant medications, it may be due to a condition known as histadelia. Histadelics have a high level of histamine in their blood that may be responsible for their depression. Multi-vitamins that contain the B vitamin folic acid may in fact make the condition worse. However, calcium supplementation is effective. It releases an amino acid, methionine, that helps to detoxify excessive histamine in the blood stream. Zinc and manganese supplementation also increases the effect with calcium. A diet that is low in protein with adequate vegetables and fruits will also help histadelics [96].

Acupuncture

Several controlled studies have shown acupuncture to have positive effects in treating depression. Acupuncture is an ancient Chinese treatment based on the belief that two types of "energies" flow in "meridians" throughout the body and that imbalances in these energies cause illness. By inserting needles in points along the meridians imbalances are corrected, restoring health. Two randomized controlled studies compared the effects of electro acupuncture and the tricycles antidepressant amitriptyline hydrochloride. After five weeks of therapy a comparison on the Hamilton Depression scale scores (from 29 to 13 and 29 to 14, respectively) indicated no significant difference between the two.

Another study, involving 241 patients receiving electroacupuncture or amitriptyline hydrochloride for six weeks also showed similar results for both treatments (depression scale scores from 35 to 8 and from 35 to 10, respectively). Follow-up of 148 patients for 2 to 4 years revealed no significant difference in the depression recurrence rate between the two groups [97].

Exercise

A large body of evidence exists relating to the positive effects that exercise has on depression. A meta-analysis of 80 studies produced an overall mean exercise effect in depression scale scores of a decrease by one-half of a standard deviation in the exercise groups than in the comparison groups. The antidepressant effect on depression from exercise occurred with all types of regular exercise, independent of sex or age, and it increased with the duration of therapy. Overall, exercise was as effective in reducing depression as psychotherapy [98].

Other Therapies:

Other alternative therapies for depression include **light therapy, therapeutic massage,** and **yoga**. Light therapy is particularly effective for people with seasonal affective disorder (SAD), a depression triggered by a lack of light and usually occurs during winter months when there are fewer hours of daylight. A typical treatment calls for sitting in front of a full-spectrum fluorescent light (one that is up to 12 times brighter than ordinary indoor light) for about two hours per day.

Recent clinical studies have also shown that therapeutic massage can ease depression. Yoga helps to reduce stress and depression by exercises such as controlled breathing and posturing that instills energy and relaxation. Using mental imagery and creative visualization during yoga encourages relaxation and improves mental outlook [99].

Biofeedback devices have also been effective in treating depression. Biofeedback is a technique of training the mind to enter relaxed states. The difference between biofeedback and a practice like yoga is that in biofeedback the individual is often connected to a device that can measure the relaxed state the brain is entering, thereby offering the individual visible control over the process.

Psychiatrist Dr. Charles Stroebel developed a device called the CAP scan that measures the different brain waves. The patient is hooked up with a number of electrodes to a computer that displays colored images representing brain wave patterns. By training the brain to control the images the individual reaches more relaxed states. Dr. Stroebel found that by hooking up depressive people to his device they can gain control over their abnormal brain wave patterns, normalize them, and feel the difference. He believes it can be a breakthrough in treating depression [100].

Meditation has been shown to be a viable option for reducing depression. In clinical studies by Jon Kabot-Zinn, Ph.D founder and director of the Stress Reduction Clinic at the University of Massachusetts Medical Center it was observed that patients that underwent training in meditation had significant reductions in depression and anxiety. Dr. Kabot-Zinn's 8 week program at the clinic teaches patients techniques of mindfulness meditation, derived from the Buddhist tradition, that is guided moment to moment awareness. Patients referred to the clinic often with chronic headaches, back pain, heart disease, cancer or AIDS to learn how to relax and cope better with the stress in their lives. However, they often leave with less severe physical symptoms, and with greater self-confidence, optimism, and assertiveness. They become less anxious, less angry and less depressed over their lives [101].

The *Harvard Mental Health Letter* (4/05) reports that meditation changes brain-wave activity. A study of Buddhists monks who were longtime meditators showed that their brain wave activity reflected large-scale coordination of neural circuits, when compared to control subjects. In another study they reported that subjects that underwent a two-month course in mindfulness meditation had persistent increased activity on the left side of the prefrontal cortex that is associated with joyful serene emotions. These positive effects were also observed four months after the meditation course ended [102].

As described in Chapter III, **hypnotherapy** has been shown to be highly effective in treating anxiety, stress and specific phobias. Hypnotherapy practices date back thousands of years, and employs the power of suggestion to heal the body or mind. Hypnotherapy uses the same techniques in treating depression. By placing the patient in a trance state by relaxing the body the hypnotherapist can positively re-program the subconscious helping the individual to alleviate depression. By suggesting relaxing techniques or using guided meditation the hypnotherapist relaxes the patient and then implants healing suggestions. Hypnotherapy has been shown to be a proven technique as an adjunct or primary therapy for a wide range of medical and psychological disorders [103].

Table 5-2
Summary of Naturopathic Treatment for Depression [60, 61, 70, 73, 79, 81, 90:]

Common Name/ (scientific name):	Acting mechanism:	Possible side effects / Interactions:
St. John's wort (*Hypericum perforatum*)	May modulate the action of Il-6, increasing adrenal hormones reducing depress-sion.	Should not be used in combination with other anti-depressants, beta-blockers, NNRTIs, seizure, heart cancer, or transplant medications.
SAMe (*S-Adenosylme-thiamine*)	Increases operation of neurotransmitters, serotonin and nor epinephrine.	Overdose can cause mania, manifested by pressured speech and a display of grandiose ideas, nausea.
Ginkgo (*Ginkgo biloba*)	Acts as anti-inflammatory, and increases oxygen in the brain.	Possible dizziness, upset stomach and mild headache.
American Ginseng (*Panax quinquefolis*)	Active compounds of ginsenosides increases blood flow in the brain.	Toxicity side effects may include diarrhea, diminished libido, earaches, headaches, high blood pressure, insomnia, rashes, nosebleeds, vomiting. No drug interactions.
Kava kava (*Piper methysticum*)	Active compounds of kavalactones modify neuro-transmitters, increases mental alertness and ele-vates mood.	Toxicity can cause skin, nail and hair discoloration, scaly skin, swollen eyes and face, muscle weakness, motor and vision problems. Negative interactions with alcohol, anti-anxiety and sleep medications (benzodiazepines).

Conclusions:

Depressive illness effects 1 in 10 Americans, appears to be growing, and effecting children at earlier ages. Percentages of MDD range from up to 2 percent of children under age 12, to 8 to 10 percent of adolescents and 10 percent of adults. The AMA indicates there are so many causes of depressive illness it can be difficult to determine.

However, there appears to be links to the function of neurotransmitters, norepinephrine, serotonin, and dopamine and the effect they have on depression. Many conditions appear to effect the levels of these neurotransmitters. Diseases such as Parkinson's can reduce the level of dopamine, some cancerous tumors can secrete serotonin causing an imbalance.

Imbalances in the functioning of the hypothalamus, adrenal, thyroid or pituitary glands may lead to depression. Illnesses such as diabetes, mononucleosis, hepatitis, pneumonia, HIV/AIDS, CFS, SLE, multiple sclerosis, Alzheimer's disease, heart disease, and stroke have been linked to depression.

Nutrient deficiencies such as the B vitamins, niacin, folic acid, vitamins A and C, calcium, iron, magnesium, selenium and zinc may contribute to depressive illness. Research has shown some 200 medications can have a side effect of depression. Medications for high blood pressure, prescription pain medications, anticonvulsant medications, and even oral contraceptives can cause depression.

American allopathic treatment for depression usually recommends antidepressant medications. Antidepressants work by altering the brain's supply of neurotransmitters, and are divided into categories based on the effect they have on the brain. Tricyclic antidepressants have been used the longest, and work by blocking the reuptake of norepinephrine, and thereby increasing the amount of it in the brain. MAOIs help to increase the levels of neurotransmitters by interfering with the production of monamine oxidase a substance found in nerve endings that breaks down neurotransmitters. SSRIs increase the brain's supply of serotonin. Atypical antidepressants may act on any of the neurotransmitters depending on the medication. Lithium is believed to operate in treating depression by slowing down the reactions of certain proteins that regulate the actions of neurotransmitters.

Antidepressant medications have a wide range of side effects and 35.9 percent of patients report adverse effects. Tricyclic antidepressants effect other neurotransmitters that help regulate certain body processes. This leads to side effects such as sleepiness, drowsiness, dry mouth, constipation, difficulty urinating, vision problems, dizziness, or a racing heart. Less common side effects are rashes, sweating, tremors, delayed ore reduced sexual functioning, weight gain, and dry eyes. Side effects of MAIOs include dizziness, changes in blood pressure, weight gain, sleepiness or insomnia, reduced sexual functioning, swollen ankles and fingers. Less frequent side effect can be dry mouth, constipation, blurred vision, and difficulty urinating. Because SSRIs target only serotonin they tend to produce fewer side effects than tricyclics or MAIOs. Side effects can include insomnia, nervousness, agitation, nausea, diarrhea, and headaches. Occasionally SSRIs can cause sexual side effects such as diminished interest in sex, arousal problems, and difficulty achieving organism. SSRIs have also been shown to speed up bone loss. A study published in the June 25, 2007 issue of the *Archives of Internal Medicine* reports an up to 60 percent greater bone loss and a twofold increase in fractures of older patients using SSRI's.

About 40 percent of people on lithium experience side effects of digestive problems like nausea, vomiting, diarrhea, and stomachaches. Excessive urination, tremors, weight gain, acne, dry skin, headaches, sleeplessness and exhaustion are also often experienced. Lithium will interact with medications such as aspirin, ibuprofen and the antibiotic tetracycline, increasing the levels of lithium in the blood to dangerous levels. And, antidepressants have reported up to 31 deaths per million prescriptions filled.

Clinical trials of psychotropic medications have shown that placebos used in the trails to be 50 percent as effective as the medications and, typically 20 to 35 percent of patients fail to respond at all to antidepressant medication.

Naturopathic, alternative or complimentary medicine has been treating mental illness for thousands of years, and its effectiveness is currently being supported by clinical trials. St. John's wort is the leading medication for depression in Germany, and sales of the herb are reported to be in excess of $200 million in the U.S. St. John's wort is believe to act similar to antidepressants by inhibiting the action of neurotransmitters. In controlled studies using St. John's wort it was found to be as effective in treating mild to moderate depression as antidepressant medications with far fewer side effects. In fact, the frequency and severity of side effects has been considered clinically insignificant, however, the FDA warns about possible drug interactions when using it in combination with other prescription medications for HIV, transplant medications, cancer treatment, and antidepressant medication.

In studies comparing SAMe with tricyclics SAMe outperformed the antidepressant medications. SAMe may act like an antidepressant or, on cell membrane structure in easing depression. SAMe also appears to have a quicker response rate than antidepressants, where patients show improvement in 7 to 14 days compared to an average of 21 days for antidepressants or St.

John's wort. However, SAMe has been shown to have a positive reaction when combined with antidepressants unlike St. John's wort.

Other herbs, although with less clinical evidence, are also believed to have positive effects in treating depression. Gingko is believed to treat depression by increasing the oxygen supply to the brain and by increasing dopamine levels. Ginseng also increases blood flow to the brain and is believed to relieve depression by its ability to reduce stress, improve mental concentration, and mental performance. Kava works as an antidepressant by acting as a central nervous system sedative targeting the limbic system which regulates moods and emotions. Lavender, and aromatic herb, has been used for a variety of mental disorders such as depression due to its ability to relax. Other essential oils are used frequently in aromatherapy for relaxation such as bergamot, clary sage, geranium, and neroli.

Nutritional treatment for depression includes limiting foods that are harmful to the body, increasing foods that are beneficial and supplementation. Traditional Chinese medicine believes depression is caused by a stagnant liver. Foods that are rich, greasy and high in saturated fats cause a stagnant liver. Limiting such foods and increasing natural foods like brown rice, whole wheat, vegetables, fruits, wheat germ, and micro-algae help cleanse the liver and provide vitamins and minerals that may be missing from the diet. Protein from turkey contains tryptophan, an amino acid that has a calming effect, protein from chicken or fish (lower in saturated fat) contain dopamine and norepinephrine. Essential Fatty acids, found in fish, marine animals and soy, have been shown to provide the brain with needed nutrients for proper functioning that prevents depression. Supplementation of B-complex vitamins (B1, B6, B12, folic acid, niacin), vitamins A and C, minerals of calcium, magnesium, selenium and zinc are necessary for proper mental health and have been used as treatments for depression.

Therapies such as acupuncture, exercise, light therapy, yoga, massage, biofeedback, meditation and hypnotherapy all offer non-drug alternatives for treatment of depression. Acupuncture has been shown to be as effective as antidepressants, and exercise has been proven to be as effective as psychotherapy in relieving depression.

Holistic Mental Health for Depression
Specific Recommendations:

Antidepressant medications that are combined with psychotherapy may be recommended for severe cases of MDD. However, antidepressant medication usually comes with a host of side effects ranging from mild to severe (life threatening) and in many cases has no effect on depression. Medication also does not appear to uncover the cause of depression. Alternative medicine has been proven to be as effective as antidepressants, without the side effects. Daily naturopathic treatment for depression could include:

- Supplements of St. John's wort, SAMe, ginkgo, ginseng and kava all have been shown to be effective treatments for depression. Herbal interventions should not be used with prescription medications and patients should always check with their physicians before combining alternative treatments with prescription medications.

- Nutritional intervention may in fact uncover causes for depression and offer a non-medication approach without side effects. A diet of natural foods such as vegetables, fruits, and whole grains, fish, and soy, and one devoid of saturated fats, red meats, greasy foods and artificial additives can help cleanse the body and mind.

- Supplements of B-complex, vitamins A, C and D, minerals of calcium, magnesium, selenium and zinc are necessary for proper nervous system function.

- Smoking and excessive caffeine also should be avoided as they interfere with the nervous system.

- Therapies such as aromatherapy, exercise, yoga, acupuncture, massage, biofeedback, meditation, and hypnotherapy may complement other therapies when used with nutritional intervention and supplementation, or herbal medicine in treating depression.

Treatment for medical conditions should always be conducted by your healthcare professional. According to the FDA only physicians are allowed to prescribe medications, and the suggestions in this book are for dietary changes and/or supplements only.

"Not everything that is faced can be changed,
but nothing can be changed until it is faced."
~ James Baldwin

"Problems cannot be solved at the same level of awareness that created
them."
~ Albert Einstein

CHAPTER VI:
Headaches & Migraines:

Headaches and migraines are most probably as old as human thought itself. The pain from a headache can range from a mild throbbing to a debilitating migraine. It is estimated that 80 million Americans experience headaches, 50 million have experienced a migraine, and 28 million suffer from migraines continually.

"Migraine" comes from the Greek word *hemicrania,* which means "half a head". The earliest known record of a headache was included in the *Ebers papyrus,* which dates to Mesopotamia in 4000 B.C. Today, the economic cost of migraines is enormous, with 150 million lost days from work or school in the U.S. and $13 million in lost productivity per year.

Women are more likely than men to suffer from migraines, as 70 percent of migraine patients are female. Migraines are more common in women than type 2 diabetes, osteoarthritis or asthma. And of the estimated 26 million women that get migraines in the U.S. only 3 to 5 percent seek preventive therapy. Thirty percent of migraine suffers have their first attack before age ten, and the disorder is very prevalent among adolescents and young adults. Poorer adolescents were found to get nearly twice as many migraines than more affluent ones. Family income may be related to stress, poor diet and less medical care, all contributing to the higher number of migraines reported in lower income families. Over $20 billion a year is spent by suffers desperate for relief from headaches and migraines [1, 2, 3, 4, 5].

A study published in *Neurology* compared first time migraine diagnoses from 1979 to 1981 and from 1989 to 1990, and found that the overall rate of migraines increased by 56 percent in women and 34 percent in men. The report suggested an increase in migraine rates may be due to increased stress levels in the population [6].

The most common types of headaches are tension headaches and migraines. Stress, irregular sleep, hormonal shifts, depression, eyestrain, and food allergies are the most common causes. And, just as in other mental disorders there is a variety of treatment options based on the cause and severity of the disorder [7].

Types of :

Headaches are usually divided into four categories; tension headaches, organic headaches, and vascular headaches that can be either cluster headaches or migraines.

Tension Headaches

Tension headaches (or muscle contraction headaches) are believed to be caused by muscle tension. Some 75 to 80 percent of the headaches people get fall into this category. And 90 percent of the population gets this type of headache from time to time. Pain is usually felt in the back of the head and neck. The pain may envelop the whole head, and feel like the head is in a vise. Along with head pain, people with these headaches often have sore shoulders and a sore neck as well. Tension headaches may last for days without relief, except for during sleep. Tension headaches usually begin during adult life, however, 10 to 20 percent of people report getting this type of headache as children and teenagers. Men and women get this type of headache about equally.

Tension headaches can be categorized as *episodic tension-type headaches* (ETTH) or *chronic tension-type headaches* (CTTH). In a recent study reported in the *Journal of The American Medical Association (JAMA)*, found the overall prevalence rate of ETTH was 38.3 percent, with the rate peaking in 30 to 39 year-olds of 42.3 percent in males and 46.9 percent in women. Prevalence rates also increased with educational levels, peaking with graduate school education of 48.5 percent for men and 48.9 percent for women. Subjects in the study reported less prevalence of CTTH (2.2%) however, CTTH subjects reported more lost workdays, 27.4 days per year compared to 8.9 days per year lost from ETTH.

Organic Headaches

Organic headaches are usually a symptom of another ailment. It could be a sign of inflammation around the brain, elevated blood pressure, a buildup of fluid around the brain, or even a brain tumor. Less than one percent of the headaches are organic, but the underlying problems may be life threatening.

Vascular Headaches

Vascular headaches gain their name from the process by which blood vessels in the head expand or dilate, and cause the pain of cluster headaches or migraine attacks.

Cluster headaches usually affects one side of the head, with severe pain around the eye. It may radiate from above the affected eye to the temple and to the jaw or gums on the same side or more rarely over half of the head. The pain may even cause the pupil of the eye on the affected side to constrict, the eye redden and occasionally droop. The cluster headache often occurs in bouts, with each lasting from four to eight weeks. The attack builds within a few minutes and lasts for a total of about 45 minutes. Several attacks may occur each day during the cluster period and may even wake the suffer from sleep. Cluster headaches appear more often in men (90 percent) than women, typically starts in their 30's, and are rare, affecting fewer than one percent of the population. They are also more frequent in the spring and fall.

Migraines are classified into *classic migraines* and *common migraines*. Up to 70 percent of migraine suffers have both types of migraines. Classic migraines are also called migraines with aura. This type is the most dramatic form of migraine. It constitutes only about 35 percent of all migraine attacks. The headache, nausea, and vomiting of this migraine attack is preceded by flashing lights or other sensory symptoms. A suffer may complain about bright stars that pass across the field of vision and even a temporary loss of sight, or double vision occurs. There may also be a tingling and pins and needles sensation in one hand or arm, or around the mouth. The tingling sensation usually starts in the fingers and gradually spreads up the arms over a period of 15 to 20 minutes. These symptoms recede after 10 to 60 minutes and are followed by headache, nausea, and vomiting. The migraine with aura usually has four stages; the prodrome stage, where symptoms start, which may include feeling tired, stiff neck, thirst, sensitivity to light and sound, irritability, and craving for sweets. The aura stage, characterized by seeing lights, tingling sensations and photosensitivity, the third stage is where the headache occurs, which is usually one-sided in the forehead or temples, and the final stage or recovery stage, where the pain subsides.

Common migraines, also called migraine without aura, differ from classic migraines where the individual does not experience the aura. Sixty-five percent of people who suffer from migraines experience this kind of migraine. It progresses in three stages, with the same symptoms; the prodrome, the headache, and the recovery stage [8, 9, 10, 11, 12].

Causes of Migraines & Headaches:

Headaches and migraines have a variety of causes and treatment should be related to the cause. The brain itself does not feel pain. Headache pain has its source in the nerves located in the muscles and blood vessels of the face, neck and scalp, in the nerves running between the back of the brain, and in the brain's blood vessels [13].

Organic Disorders

About ten percent of individuals seeking help for headaches have some organic disorder for which the headache is a symptom. However, only one percent of those seeking help for headaches have a brain tumor. Headache is rarely the first sign of a brain tumor. Usually a tumor is accompanied by or preceded vomiting, personality changes, noticeable changes in mental functioning, including difficulty in concentration, drowsiness, seizures, or fainting. The headache pain feels like a tight band squeezing the head, but there is also a persistent pain that may be concentrated in one area that seems to build. The pain from a brain tumor headache may wake a person from sleep, and the pain increases, whenever the person coughs, strains, or suddenly moves the head [14].

The pain of a brain tumor comes from the pressure of the tumor pressing against meninges, or the brain covering, within the skull, or against may arteries or sinuses. Because the brain feels no pain, the tumor must grow quite a bit for the body to feel pain. Before this happens the tumor's pressure is likely to produce other symptoms, which is why a headache is one of the last signs of a brain tumor When changes in personality are accompanied by increasing headache pain medical intervention should be pursued [15, 16].

Other organic conditions of headaches can include hemorrhaging into the layers of the meninges, or into the brain itself, ruptured aneurysms, meningitis, temporal arthritis, or head injuries. Problems with muscles or joints of the jaw can cause headaches (temporomandibular joint - TMJ). Eye problems such as glaucoma, an eye disease that is caused by increasing pressure in the eyeball. As glaucoma develops, an individual frequently experiences acute throbbing pain around or behind the eye and in the forehead. The pain is felt in other areas in the head so that it feels like a headache.

Injuries to the head can result in chronic headaches. Most postconcussional syndrome symptoms include headache that may be caused by reduced cerebral blood flow and excessive release of excitatory amino acids that are some of the same mechanisms that are believed to be related to the development of migraines. Headaches have also been associated with obstructive sleep apnea (OSA). Patients with OSA report an 80 percent reduction in waking up with headaches when treated for their OSA by continuous positive airway pressure or uvulopalatopharyngoplasty [17, 18, 19].

Causes of Tension Headaches

Tension (or muscle-contraction) headaches can either be acute or chronic. Acute tension headaches are temporary, specific responses to particular events. They can be caused by a stressful event, and are usually responsive to rest, relaxation and over-the-counter medications. Chronic tension headaches are frequent, at least twice a week, and extend up to seven days a week. People who suffer from chronic tension headaches will usually wake up with a headache, or develop one early in the day. The pain of a chronic tension headache is usually found in the forehead and the back of the head and neck. Along with head pain people usually experience sore shoulders and a sore neck. These types of headaches can be caused by staying in the same position, sitting, reading, typing, or driving, for a long period of time. This may cause reduced blood supply in the area, causing metabolic wastes to accumulate that the blood stream would normally wash away. Stress may be an underlying cause of the tension as well.

Chronic tension headaches are often associated with depression and sleep disturbance. This implies a dysfunction of the serotonergic system, which controls sleep, the sensation of dull pain, emotions, and the sense of well-being. Often when chronic tension headache suffers wake up with a headache it may be the result of uninhibited hours of sleep when distressful feelings that have been ignored throughout the day finally come to the surface. The body reacts to those feelings by contracting its muscles protectively, and the individual awakes with a feeling of depression and headache [20].

Chronic tension headaches may also be the result of other physical factors. Arthritis, neck abnormalities or nerve damage can all lead to headache pain.

If the joints of the neck develop arthritis the muscles around the joints instinctively contract in order to "split" the pain. Unfortunately this makes the pain worse. If the arthritis causes a spinal disk to degenerate it may press on a nerve that extends from the spinal cord. This pinched nerve is not fully functioning. If the nerve is in the upper cervical area (neck area) it may refer pain to the head. Neck abnormalities are also possible origins of a muscle contraction or tension headache. Injuries to the neck, like whiplash, a spinal tumor, or congenital (present from birth) deformities may put pressure on a nerve, causing pain and the consequent muscle contraction response to it [21].

Causes of Sinus Headaches

Sinus headaches are due to the inflammation of the sinus cavities called sinusitis. Acute sinus headaches are caused by an infection. Symptoms include tenderness in the sinus area, headache, fever, and a greenish yellow discharge from throat or nose. Chronic sinus headaches are also caused by inflammation, but there is no infection. There may be headache, but it is usually accompanied by a feeling of stuffiness, or fullness, instead of pain, and there is no fever. Migraines are often confused with sinus headaches due to the location of the pain [22].

Causes of Migraines

Migraines are estimated to affect 8 to 10 percent of all men and 18 to 20 percent of all women at some point in their lives. The disorder affects more women then men (up to 75 percent are women), and the onset of migraines break down to 25 percent getting their first migraine by age ten, 56 percent by age 13, 75 percent by age 30, and 90 percent by age 40. Migraines are known as vascular headaches because they involve the blood vessels in the face, head and neck. Sometimes they become unnaturally narrowed (constricted) other times they become abnormally widened (dilated). If the blood vessels in the head are constricted there is an accumulation of chemical irritants within the blood vessels, since a normal flow of blood is not pulsing through to wash the irritants away.

An excess of neurokinin, a substance similar to a material found in wasp venom, has been found in migraine suffers when experiencing headache pain. The vasoconstriction seems to set off the opposite reaction, vasodilatation in the blood vessels on the surface of the brain and scalp. This corresponds to the throbbing, painful stage of the migraine, that seems as though the head might burst from an excess of blood. Part of the pain does in fact come from the pressure on nerves in the blood vessels being dilated to an unnatural width [23, 24].

There are several theories as to what sets off this process of **vasoconstriction** and **vasodilatation,** causing migraines. Changes in levels of serotonin may cause this change in the blood vessels. Serotonin levels have been found to be high in the brain before a migraine, and low during the migraine. Serotonin has the effect of constricting blood vessels, and when the level drops in the brain, just before the migraine comes on, there is also a drop in mood, characterized by depression. Migraine suffers often have a family history of depression and migraine attacks. Serotonin has a nitrogen containing substance in it called an amine. Amines also comprise noradrenaline, histamine, and dopamine, all of which affect blood vessels, sleep patterns and mood. Migraine suffers find that foods high in certain amines (such as chocolate, cheese and alcohol) set off a headache, along with a period of depression that precedes it. Another amine, tyramine, causes blood vessels to start the constriction process and release prostaglandins that further affect blood vessels by causing them to expand. This sensitivity to amines are often found in migraine suffers to where they seemingly have lower defenses to these chemicals found in foods. Another over-sensitivity that may cause a migraine is an individual's over reaction to stress which produces adrenaline, which in turn can cause a headache [25].

Differences in Brain Structure

Harvard Medical School investigators using magnetic resonance imaging (MRI) found structural differences between the brains of those suffering from migraines and those not. The MRI's showed thickening of a specific area of the brain related to the communication of sensory processing called the somatosensory cortex (SSC). Other studies have shown similar differences in the cortex thickness in patients with multiple sclerosis and Alzheimer's Disease. Researchers believe that individuals may be born with these cortical differences making them more susceptible to migraines later in life. However, they did comment they were not entirely sure if migraines cause brain changes, or if the brain differences cause migraines. The studies do show that there are structural differences and that the SSC plays an important role in migraines [26].

The reason women may get more migraines then men may also have to with the fact that there brains are "wired" differently. A new study suggests that the reason may be that their brains are faster to activate the cascading waves of activity thought to cause migraine pain as well as other migraine symptoms. Advances in brain imaging technology now suggest that migraines may start as a result of brain excitability. People with migraines show dramatic waves of brain activity that spread across the surface of the brain, known as cortical spreading depression (CSD). CSD is thought to trigger not only the severe pain associated with migraines, but also the visual symptoms, dizziness, and difficulty concentrating, often associated with migraines. Researchers found that the strength required to stimulate the CSD was 2 to 3 times higher in males than in females. They also believe that there are many factors that reduce the threshold of CSD such as genes, hormones and environmental triggers like stress, diet, and changes in sleep patterns [27].

Nutritional Deficiencies

Another factor that is believed to be responsible for half of all migraines is related to magnesium levels in the body. Magnesium helps to regulate serotonin levels in the brain, and it has been found that migraine suffers lack this essential mineral. Without magnesium serotonin levels are not properly regulated, blood vessels do not retain their proper size, inflammation sets in, and a migraine develops. Magnesium also helps other chemicals in the body that regulate dilation and constriction. Research conducted by Dr. Alexander Mauskop, at the New York Headache Center, has shown that patients respond positively to magnesium therapy. Magnesium taken by supplements or injection had the effect of stopping the migraines in its tracks [28].

Overactive Hypothalamus

Another theory as to the cause of migraines involves the **hypothalamus**. The hypothalamus gland is located behind the eyes, above the pituitary gland in the center of the brain. It is responsible for body functions such as hunger, sleep cycles, the timing of menstrual cycles and other hormonal secretions. It also communicates with the brain stem, which contains the body's pain fighting system. This communication channel may be oversensitive to pain with people that suffer from migraines [29].

Hypoglycemia

Hypoglycemia may lead to headaches and migraines. Hypoglycemia is caused when the pancreas is overactive, producing too much insulin (the opposite of diabetes, where too little insulin is produced). So much insulin is produced that the body's blood sugar drops to 40 to 50 mg (70 to 110 mg is normal) percent. Too much glucose (which is converted by insulin) leaves the blood vessels for the body's tissues. There may be a greater degree of hypoglycemia after eating, and especially after drinking alcohol, or eating foods that contain sugar. This drop in blood sugar is experienced as an emergency by the body, similar to when the body is under severe stress. In trying to get the glucose level back up the body stimulates the adrenal glands which produces catecholamines. These chemical neurotransmitters constrict the blood vessels to get blood traveling through the body more quickly in order to bring what little blood sugar is left to the body's tissues.

The catecholamines also raise the body temperature, blood pressure, and pulse rate and produce headaches, a feeling of panic, irritability and despair. The blood vessel constriction can't last forever, so the opposite effect is triggered by the production of prostaglandins. The blood vessels become dilated which produces the throbbing pain of a migraine. Studies have shown when people susceptible to migraines are given a shot of insulin, they develop a migraine, however people who do not get migraines did not experience a migraine when getting even a double dose of insulin [30].

Food Allergies

In addition to the effects of sugar causing migraines in hypoglycemics, many people have specific food allergies that have been shown to cause headaches and migraines. These food triggers include: pork; game and organ meats (including liver, kidney, and brains); smoked and cured, aged and packaged meat (like corned beef, cold cuts, salami, hot dogs, ham and sausage); herring, caviar, and smoked fish; vinegar; pickled and fermented foods; aged cheese (like cheddar, Brie, and Gruyere); products high in yeasts and tyramines (doughnuts, coffee cakes, and breads); chocolate; sugar and all products made with processed sugar or corn syrup; yogurt; the pods of lima beans, navy beans, and peas; flavor enhancers such as MSG (monosodium glutamate); caffeine; and alcoholic beverages, especially red wine.

Studies on food allergies related to the cause of migraine range from 30 to 93 percent responsible for the migraine. Specific foods causing migraines and their percentage in causing (top 10) are: cow's milk (67%), eggs (60%), chocolate (55%), wheat (52%), oranges (52%), benzoic acid (35%), cheese (32%), tomatoes (32%), tartrazine (30%), and rye (30%). Aspartame, the sugar substitute in the sweetener *NutraSweet,* has been found to trigger headache in as many as 10 percent of migraine sufferers [31, 32, 33].

Digestion Disorders

Many health-oriented doctors believe headaches and migraines originate from the stomach. Migraines can be caused by excess starches and sugars in the diet. Wrong food combinations, overeating, and junk foods will cause fermentation in the intestines and stomach. This causes gas, which enters the blood and causes irritation on the nerves and brain, and causes headaches. Pressure in the head and in the temples could mean there is stomach problems. Throbbing pain often results from congestion in the liver, spleen, or digestive tract [34].

Environmental Factors

Smoking: Smokers have high incidence of migraines. Nicotine in tobacco is a vasoconstrictor that the body becomes dependent on. As the body needs ever higher amounts to keep the blood vessels constricted rebound effects occur leading to headaches. In addition smokers have large amounts of carbon monoxide and carboxyhemoglobin in their blood, substances that displace oxygen and cause a lack of oxygen in the brain. Lack of oxygen causes blood vessels to dilate in an attempt to carry more blood to the brain, which may trigger a headache [35].

A great many migraine suffers develop migraines due to environmental triggers. The most common being related to allergy toxins. People susceptible to allergies from pollen and molds can also get migraines when their blood vessels become inflamed and dilate from the reaction to the allergens. Environmental toxins that can lead to migraine attacks include pollen, dust (dust mites), pets (especially cats), gas stove emissions, household cleaners, perfume, cosmetics, fabric cleaners, hairspray, air fresheners, cigarette smoke, car exhausts, smog, pesticides, and natural gas.

Some people develop migraines due to changes in the weather. Certain types of weather such as in the springtime, or hot humid days of summer, or the onset of storms can increase the frequency and severity of migraines. Springtime encourages migraines because of the proliferation of allergens in the air. The heat and humidity of summer encourages mold growth, the release of grass pollens, and the proliferation of heavy smog. Sudden rainstorms cause a drop in barometric pressure. Along with a drop in barometric pressure the ratio of positive to negative ions in the air changes. An increase in the positive ions carries with them more allergens that attach themselves to the positive ions [36].

Sleep Disturbance

Studies in the journal *Headache* found that most women that suffer from migraines report that they complain about sleep problems as well. Eighty percent of 147 women in a study reported that they were tired when they awoke. In another study, when participants received behavioral sleep instructions had a significant reduction in migraine headache and frequency and intensity. Researchers explain that a sleep disturbances interrupts REM sleep. Normal REM produces serotonin and dopamine, the feel good neurotransmitters in the brain. A decrease in these neurotransmitters are associated with poor sleep or sleep problems. Migraine suffers often awake with a migraine because REM sleep is the most powerful just before awakening, and insufficient REM causing a lower level of serotonin and dopamine initiates the migraine [37].

Medications

Certain prescription medications have caused migraines. Agents used for treating high blood pressure like minoxidil or reserpine can cause migraines. Medications for treating heart disease (nitrates) and arthritis (indomethacin) have caused migraines. Estrogen used in birth control pills and hormonal replacement therapy cause migraines in some women [38].

Genetics

Most headache researchers believe migraines are a hereditary disease. About 70 percent of migraine sufferers have a family history of migraines. Recently researchers have identified a chromosome, chromosome 19, that they believe is a genetic link to migraines. The incidence of migraines is especially high if both parents have suffered from migraines [39].

Allopathic Treatment for Headaches and Migraines:

For tension and migraine headaches that occur once a week or less, over-the-counter (OTC) pain relievers can be effective. They include; aspirin, acetaminophen, a combination of aspirin or acetaminophen and caffeine, nonsteroidal anti-inflammatory drugs, such as ibuprofen and naproxen sodium. If these medications fail to produce results, prescription painkillers may work. All of these medications carry warnings of side effects from stomach ulcers to chest tightness, and dangerous interactions with other drugs. Overuse of both prescription medications and over-the-counter painkillers can lead to drug rebound headaches. When this happens, a once-effective drug no longer produces results, and when the dose wears off, another, worse headache appears [40].

Medications to treat migraines fall into two larger categories: ***abortive drugs*** to stop migraines in progress, and ***prophylactic drugs*** to prevent future ones from striking.

Abortive Drugs:

Corticosteroids: Prednisone and other corticosteroids work by dampening the body's inflammation response. They are used for very long-lasting migraines that do not respond to other treatments. Side effects include insomnia, anxiety, and agitation. Depending on the drug, the corticosteroids may be given orally or by injection. These drugs have a large number of serious side effects if used for long periods of time.

Ergot derivatives: *Cafergot, Migranal, Relpax,* and other drugs in this family are derived from a plant fungus. They are felt to help with migraines by constricting the blood vessels in the brain. Their potential side effects include nausea, vomiting, muscle cramps, high blood pressure, slow heartbeat, and vertigo. They can be taken orally, by injection, or by a suppository.

Opioids or narcotics: *Percocet, Vicodin, Demerol,* and other powerful painkillers are used for more serious migraines that do not respond to first line treatment. Side effects include dizziness, sedation, vomiting, irritability, and perspiration. There is also the risk of dependency and addiction.

NSAIDS: these are the nonsteroidal anti-inflammatory drugs prescribed for arthritis and other painful diseases. Ibuprofen (*Advil, Motrin*), anaprox or naprelan, (*Aleve*), naproxen (*Naprosyn*), ketoprofen(*Orudis*), Nabumetone (*Relafen*), other NSAIDS and over-the-counter versions of aspirin, have long been used for the treatment of migraines. Side effects include urinary track infections, diarrhea, nausea, heartburn, ringing in the ears (tinnitus), and stomach bleeding.

Triptans: A newer treatment for migraines, Triptans work by encouraging the action of serotonin. They can be taken orally, by nasal spray or injection. Amerge, Imitrex, Maxalt, and Zomig are members of this family of medications. Potential side effects include feeling warm, muscle weakness, shortness of breath, chest pain, and anxiety. Heart disease patients should not take Triptans because of their effect in constricting blood vessels. The FDA has issued a warning that triptans should not be used with depression and mood disordered drugs such as SSRIs or SNRIs. When combined with these drugs a life-threatening condition called serotonin syndrome may occur. Symptoms can include rapid heart beat, changes in blood pressure, increased body temperature, overactive reflexes, nausea, vomiting, and diarrhea.

Combination Drugs: These include *Fiorinal* (butalbital, caffeine and aspirin), *Fioricet* and *Esgic* (butalbital, caffeine, and acetaminophen), and *Midrin* (isometheptene, dichloralphenazone, and acetaminophen). Potential side effects include somnolence, worsening of headaches with frequent use, and, with the exception of Midrin, dependency with addiction [36,37,38]. Combination of caffeine with other natural substances has been reported in medical literature in more than the last 100 years. The <u>*American Family Physician*</u> first published in 1883, reports treatment of headaches with guarana, cannabis indica, and citrate of caffeine [41, 42].

Prophylatic Drugs:

Antidepressants: Tricyclic antidepressants (TCAs) are known to block the re-absorption of serotonin. TCAs are not considered to be the first choice in migraine preventive therapy, but may be useful for some patients with coexisting migraine and tension headaches. Amitriptyline (*Elavil*), Nortriptyline (*Pamelor*), Doxepin (*Sinequan*), and Protriptyline (*Vivactil*) are some of the more effective antidepressants used for migraines. Side effects of antidepressants include dry mouth, constipation, somnolence, anxiety, irregular heartbeat, elevated blood pressure, blurred vision, sexual dysfunction, and weight gain.

Some of the newer antidepressants such as the serotonin reuptake inhibitors (SSRIs) appear to act more specifically on serotonin receptors. Like TCAs they take two to three weeks before there is any therapeutic effect. SSRIs that have been used for migraine treatment include Fluoxetine (*Prozac*), sertraline, (*Zoloft)* and Paroxetine *(Paxil)* Their side effects include nausea, insomnia, agitation, weight loss, and sexual dysfunction. Other antidepressants that have some effect are Bupropion *(Wellbutrin),* and Trazodone *(Desyrel).* They have similar side effects however, *Wellbutrin* may also produce seizure, and *Desyrel* is not recommended for male patients as it can produce priapism (penis discomfort).

Antiseizure medication: Medications like divalproex sodium (*Depakote)* and other medications used to prevent seizures have been used to treat migraines. These drugs suppress excessive excitation of all brain cells, which may include areas of the brain affected by a migraine. And are believed to increase the levels of GABA, which is a contributor to migraine development. Side effects of these medications include weight gain, loss of hair, bruising, nausea, and potential damage to the liver and pancreas. gabapentin (*Neurontin)* and topiramate (*Topamax)* are other anticonvulsants being used for the treatment of pain associated with migraines, with fewer side effects.

Beta-blockers: Propranolol *(Inderal)*, metoprolol *(Lopressor)*, timolol (*Blocadren)*, nadolol (*Corzide)*, and other members of this family of drugs are best known as medications for heart problems and high blood pressure. The beta-blockers help to relax blood vessels and interfere with the catecholamine hormones that attempt to constrict the blood vessels. Potential side effects include dizziness, slow heartbeat, depression, and fatigue, and should not be used by patients with asthma.

Calcium channel blockers: Like the beta-blockers, these drugs were designed to treat elevated blood pressure and heart problems. These drugs work by interfering with calcium, which constricts blood vessels. However, Verapamil *(Calan)* and other calcium channel blockers are not highly effective and side effects such as constipation, congestive heart failure, fluid retention, shortness of breath, blurred vision, flushing and impotence.

MAO inhibitors: Nardil (phenelzine) and other members of this family of drugs are primarily intended to treat depression. They are also used for migraines, especially severe attacks and for chronic daily headaches. Unfortunately, MAOIs can cause a number of side effects such as weight gain, dry mouthy, insomnia, and constipation. Overdoses can lead to tremor, manic behavior and other psychotic problems. They also interact with a number of foods and other drugs negatively.

Botox: Or Botulinum toxin type A was originally developed for the treatment of involuntary forceful blinking. Then it was noticed that it was effective for wrinkles around the eyes. This in turn led to the observation that migraines improved when Botox was used. It appears to relieve frontal head pain for as long as three months with one application [43, 44, 45].

Table 6-1
Summary of Allopathic Treatment for Migraine & Headache [35, 36,37]:

Drug: (Brand name)	Acting mechanism:	Possible side effects:
Prednisone	Anti-inflammatory steroid.	Insomnia, mood changes, prolong use may cause eye problems.
Ergot Derivatives: **Ergotamine tartrate** (*Cafergot*) **Dihydroergotamine Mesylate** (*Migranal*) **Eletriptan hydro-bromide** (*Relpax*)	Helps to narrow widening blood vessels in the head.	Nausea, vomiting, upset stomach, restlessness, insomnia, numbness, irregular heartbeat. May cause dependence or rebound headaches if used for an extended period of time.
Opioids: **Acetaminophen,** **Oxycodone hydrochloride** (*Percocet*), **Hydrochloride bitartrate,** **Acetaminophen** (*Vicodin*), **Meperidine hydrochloride** (*Demerol*)	Reduces pain and fever.	Dizziness, drowsiness, nausea., vomiting, sweating. Should not be taken with MAO Inhibitors.
NSAIDS: **Ibuprofen** (*Advil*) (*Motrin*), **Ketoprofen** (*Orudis*) **Nabumetone** (*Relafen*) **Naproxen** (*Aleve*)	Blocks an enzyme that produces prostaglandins, and reduces swelling, pain, and fever.	Urinary track infections, diarrhea, nausea, heartburn, ringing in the ears (tinnitus), and stomach bleeding.
Triptans: **Frovatriptan** (*Frova*) **Naratriptan** (*Amerge*) **Rizatriptan** (*Maxalt*) **Sumatriptan** (*Imitrex*) **Zolmitriptan** (*Zomig*)	Constricts blood vessels in brain. May also block pain receptors.	Flushing, numbness, sightedness, weakness, drowsiness, dizziness.
Antidepressants: **Almotriptan** (*Axert*)	Stops abnormal dilation of blood vessels in the head.	Dry mouth, headache, nausea, sleepiness, stroke.

Anti-seizure: **Divalproex** *(Depakote)* **Gabapentin** *(Neurontin)* **Topiramate** *(Topamax)*	Suppress excessive excitation of all brain cells. Increases the levels of GABA,	Weight gain, loss of hair, bruising, nausea, and potential damage to the liver and pancreas.
Beta Blockers: **Propranolol** *(Inderal)*, **Metoprolol** *(Lopressor)*, **Nadolol** *(Corgard)*	Relax blood vessels and interfere with the catecholamine hormones that attempt to constrict the blood vessels.	Dizziness, slow heartbeat, depression, and fatigue, and should not be used by patients with asthma.
Calcium Channel Blockers: **Verapamil** *(Calan, Isoptin)*	Interferes with calcium absorption that may constrict blood vessels.	Constipation, congestive heart failure, fluid retention, shortness of breath, blurred vision, flushing and impotence.
MAO Inhibitors: **Phenelzine sulfate** *(Nardil)*	Increases function of neuro-transmitters.	Weight gain, dry mouthy, insomnia, and constipation. Overdoses can lead to tremor, manic behavior and other psychotic problems.
Botox:	Injections around forehead and eyes relieves pain.	Redness bruising and infection at injection site. Dizziness, difficulty swallowing, respiratory infections.
Combination Drugs: **Isometheptene-** **Acetaminophen-** **Dichloralphenazone** *(Amindrine, Isocom, Midchlor, Midrin,* **Butalbital-** **Acetaminophen-Caffeine** *(Esgic, Fioricet)*	Relieves tension, decreases pain, widens blood vessels, relaxes body.	Dizziness, drowsiness, nausea., fever, irregular heart beat.

Naturopathic Treatment for Headaches and Migraines:

Naturopathic treatment or what is termed alternative medicine or complementary medicine emphasizes eliminating those things that cause or make the body vulnerable to recurrent headaches, recognizing that the pain is an important way for the body to alert us to trouble. The naturopathic approach to curing headaches and migraines looks into the cause first. A naturopathic physician would first conduct a physical exam, coupled with a dietary and nutritional evaluation and allergy tests. Hormone-related causes and bowel toxemia would also be considered. In the investigation, diet receives careful scrutiny.

Certain foods have been shown to bring on tension or migraine headaches in susceptible people. Such foods include: aged cheese, nuts, citrus fruits, chocolate, hot dogs, red wine, and coffee and caffeine in other beverages. Some of these foods are believed to influence headaches by containing substances that affect blood vessels in the head. Other foods may cause allergic reactions that contribute to pain. Sugar may contribute to headaches by causing wild fluctuations of blood sugar levels. Supplements such as magnesium or niacin, that have an effect on the proper functioning of blood vessels and quercetin, which can help block inflammation, are recommended [46].

Dr. Mauskop's Triple Therapy

Dr. Alexander Mauskop, director of the New York Headache Center, has developed a headache and migraine treatment program he calls "triple therapy". This therapy consists of three natural substances: **magnesium, riboflavin** (B2) and a herb, **feverfew**. Reports of using magnesium for treatment of migraines dates back over seventy years, when it was noticed that deficiencies caused headaches.

Recent studies showing the low levels of magnesium in the blood of migraine suffers supported this connection. Dr. Mauskop found that giving migraine patients intravenous injections of magnesium would often relieve their attacks within 15 minutes. He found that magnesium helps keep the blood vessels in the brain properly toned and open, allowing blood to flow freely, prevents arteries from going into sudden spasm, and it helps platelets from sticking together to keep the blood flowing [47].

Riboflavin is a B vitamin that plays several essential roles in the body such as: the release of energy from the carbohydrates, protein, and fats, normal growth, helps in the manufacture of red blood cells, the regulation of hormones, and the conversion of tryptophan into niacin. Migraine suffers appear to need more riboflavin than others due to a possible defect in the function of mitochondria, the energy generators of the cells in the body. A 1998 study found that riboflavin supplementation was superior to placebos in reducing the number of migraine headaches. A Belgian headache study compared the effect of riboflavin to aspirin in migraine incidence. In the study, 49 people took 400 mg of riboflavin per day for three months, while another 23 people took one aspirin per day. Migraine severity was found to decrease by 70 percent by the group using riboflavin, while the group taking aspirin showed no effect [48, 49].

Feverfew, *Tanacetum parthenium,* is a herb that has a long history of use in healing headaches. Unlike vitamins and minerals that were only "discovered" in the past century, "modern" reports of feverfew date back to 1649, where a British herbalist noted that the herb was a good remedy for 'all pains in the head". In 1772, physician John Hill in his book *The Family Herbal,* stated, "In the worst headache this herb exceeds whatever else is known." The ancient Greeks were reported to use the herb for swelling, inflammation, and menstrual problems. Unfortunately, like most herbal remedies it was all but forgotten by the 1950s as the medical community was being bombarded by new pharmaceuticals. However, in the late 1970s a report of a women who used feverfew to banish her migraine headaches appeared in British newspapers, and studies on the herb were renewed.

Several controlled clinical studies in the 1980s and 1990s support feverfew's ability to successfully reduce the symptom and number of attacks of migraines. One study, reported in the *British Medical Journal* in 1985 stated of 270 migraine suffers in the study, 72 percent of them had decreased frequency and severity of attacks when taking feverfew daily. A double-blind controlled study in 1988 reported by the British medical journal *The Lancet* confirmed feverfew's effectiveness in treating migraines and headaches. Feverfew is believed to be effective in treatment of migraines due to parthenolide, a substance in the herb that helps dampen the inflammation process associated with migraines. It may also mitigate the effects of histamine and arachidonic acid that contributes to headaches and their symptoms.

Feverfew is also believed to inhibit the secretion of serotonin from platelets, decrease blood vessel response to vasconstrictors (adrenaline, acetylcholine, bradykinin, prostaglandins, histamine, and serotonin), and it inhibits the production of inflammatory biochemicals (prostaglandins, leukotrienes, and thromboxanes). Side effects of feverfew are few and very mild. Minor mouth sores and gastrointestinal upset were reported in 8 percent of users, and rare allergic reactions and rapid heartbeat have also been reported. Because of its centuries-long use the herb is considered nontoxic. Recommended dosage of feverfew is 50 mg in capsule form, and 1 to 2 grams during an attack. Herbalists recommend daily doses of feverfew to reduce the frequency of migraines [50, 51, 52, 53, 54, 55].

Dr. Mauskop's triple therapy for migraine relief consists of: 300 to 400 mg of magnesium, 400 mg of riboflavin (B2), and 100 mg of feverfew per day. He suggests breaking the total dosage in half, and taking it in two doses with meals. There is a product called *Migra-Lieve*, that has all three supplements in it, in the right amounts, requiring the individual to take only two pills a day. There are few side effects with this therapy. Riboflavin is a water soluble vitamin, meaning the body excretes excesses of the vitamin, with no side effects. It is possible to take in too much magnesium, and over-dose symptoms include drowsiness, breathing difficulty, weakness, and lethargy, and may interfere with calcium absorption. Feverfew can interfere with the normal ability of the blood to clot. People on anticoagulant medications or that have blood problems should use caution in taking feverfew. However, these side effects are rare with the recommended doses in Dr. Mauskop's program [56].

Nutritional Therapies:

Other nutritional therapies that have been studied in migraine treatment include the use of cayenne pepper, quercetin and niacin. Cayenne pepper *Capsicum frutescens,* contain the active ingredient capsaicin, that gives hot peppers its hot , pungent taste. It is believed that capsaicin depletes substance P in sensory nerves after an initial stimulation of substance P release, and acts as a potent inhibitor of platelet aggregation and thereby relieves pain. Capsaicin may be a better treatment in preventing an attack then relieving one in progress, based on its ability to promote the release of substance P.

Quercetin is a bioflavonoid that helps to promote cell health and inhibits many of the pathways of inflammation. It is also believe to act as protection against foods that may induce migraine attacks. Niacin, due to its vasodilatory effects, has long been recommended in the popular literature for treatment of migraine headaches. The use was studied in the 1940s, and researchers found that intravenous injections of up to 50 mg resulted in relief of symptoms in 17 out of 21 patients. These results were confirmed in other studies [57].

Other essential vitamins and minerals that are recommended for headache and migraine control include vitamin A, B_5, B_6, B_{12}, vitamin C, vitamin E, potassium, iron, iodine and zinc. Vitamin A heals the mucous membranes, however overdoses can cause headaches (over 50,000 IUs a day). It should not be taken when taking prescription acne medication like tetracycline that can lead to an overdose and headaches.

The B vitamins helps the body cope with stress, aids in intermediary metabolism, and the metabolism of sugar and carbohydrates. B vitamins are depleted by caffeine, birth control pills, alcohol, and stress. Headache suffers often have vitamin Bs deficiencies. Vitamin C with bioflavonoids constricts and cleans veins, and vitamin E increases oxygen in the blood. Minerals such as potassium, iron, iodine, and zinc are essential for proper nervous system functioning [58, 59, 60].

Essential Fatty Acids

Essential fatty acids (EFAs) through their influence on the production of the "good" prostaglandins, that reduce the blood vessel spasm and inflammation common in migraines, may help reduce the frequency of headaches. EPA (eicosapentaenoic acid), an omega-3 fatty acid, directs the cascade of chemical alterations that lead from the raw fatty acid to the final prostaglandin products toward the production of good prostaglandins by blocking the step that produces arachidonic acid, the forerunner of all the "bad" messengers. To increase this production of good prostaglandins there must be a balance between two EFAs, linoleic acid (GLA) found in products like evening primrose oil and EPA found in cold water fish like salmon, mackerel, or sardines. The ratio of GLA and EPA should be 1:4, which can be achieved by taking 500 mg of evening primrose oil, 1,000 mg of EPA fish oil, and 200 IUs of vitamin E [61]. Tocopherol vitamin E has also been used for headaches. Supplemental vitamin E has also been used to relieve headaches during menstrual disorders [62, 63].

Valerian

Herbal therapy treatment of headaches and migraines use calming, regulating and restoring herbs. Tension-headache sufferers can benefit from herbs that soothe the body and mind Valerian *Valeriana officinalis,* has been used for centuries in folk medicine to treat headaches and migraines. Valerian has well documented sedative properties and anti-spasmodic properties, that may not cure migraines, but offer some relief in the discomfort associated with them. Teas made from chamomile or passionflower help relax stiff muscles in the head and neck, reducing pressure on the blood vessels. [64].

Ephedra

Ephedra, or ma-huang (*Ephedra sinica*), a Chinese herb, has been used in traditional Chinese medicine for over 2,000 years. It has been used to treat bronchial asthma, colds and flu, chills, nasal congestion, aching joints, and bones, cough and wheezing, edema and headache. Ephedra's alkaloids ephedrine and pseudoephedrine stimulate the central nervous system and heart muscle, dilate bronchial tubes, and elevate blood pressure.

Ephedra also has diuretic and anti-inflammatory effects that may help relieve headaches. Side effects of Ephedra include insomnia, motor disturbances, high blood pressure, glaucoma, impaired cerebral circulation, and urinary disturbances. Ephedra containing products should not be used by people that have hypertension, heart disease, thyroid disease, diabetes, or anyone taking MAOIs [65, 66].

Skullcap

Skullcap, *Scutellaria lateriflora,* is a member of the mint family and can be found in the moist soils in eastern North America. also called mad-dog skullcap, it was originally used to treat rabies. It has been found to be a nerve tonic and sedative for relieving anxiety, neuralgia, and insomnia.

In Chinese medicine it has been used to treat fevers, colds, high blood pressure, hypertension, insomnia, intestinal inflammation and headaches. Caution should be taken to use pure forms of American skullcap, some commercial products mix it with pink skullcap *Teucrium canadense,* that has been reported to be linked to liver damage [67, 68].

Willow Bark

Willow bark is considered a natural aspirin. It is derived from the inner bark of several trees from the Salix family: white willow *Salix alba,* crack willow *Salix fragilis,* purple willow *Salix purpurea,* violet willow *Salix daphnoides,* and bay willow *Salix pentandra.* For more than 2,000 years people in the northern hemisphere used willow bark as a wash for external ulcers, and internally to reduce fevers, relieve aches, pains, rheumatism, arthritis, and headaches.

In 1763, a Dr. Stone of London recommended willow bark to the medical community for the treatment of fevers. In the 1890s the Bayer Company was in search of a substitute to replace wintergreen and black birch oil, then used to relieve pain, because they were too toxic. Bayer researchers synthesized a derivative from the Salix family, acetylsalicylic acid that is known today as aspirin.

Willow bark compounds are oxidized in the liver to produce salicylic acid. It has pain relieving effects like aspirin, but with fewer side effects. Willow bark is available in dried bark form, powdered, capsules, and tea. Willow bark is high in tannins that could possibly damage the liver and like aspirin, could cause stomach ulcers if taken in high enough doses [69, 70].

Thyme

Thyme *Thymus vulgaris,* is commonly used as a culinary herb, but it has also been used to treat tension headaches when used in a tea. Hot thyme tea has been used to treat insomnia, cramps, whooping cough, and diarrhea. It is believed that the plant's aromatic essential oils are responsible for its therapeutic actions, which are largely antiseptic and antispasmodic.

The chemical constituents thymol and carvacrol account for most of thyme's essential oils, and are both strong antiseptics that can quickly soothe congested mucous membranes and calm throbbing muscles and nerves. The dried herb, made from crushed leaves and flower tops is used for teas in relieving the pain for tension headaches [71].

Other Herbs:

Less studied herbs that have been used to treat headaches and migraines include *doug quai, ginkgo* and *quercetin.* **Doug quai,** *Angelica sinensis,* is used to prevent migraine attacks by blocking the production of prostaglandins and has anti-inflammatory properties. Side effects of doug quai may be a mild laxative effect, and people on prescription blood-thinners should avoid this herb. Recommended doses are 500 to 1,000 mg, per day. **Ginkgo,** *Ginkgo biloba,* is believed to help migraines by enhancing cerebral circulation. Ginkgo increases the body's production of adenosine triphosphate (ATP), a compound that is a main source of energy at the cellular level. This activity has been shown to boost the brain's metabolism of glucose for energy to increase its electrical activity. Ginkgo flavonoids act specifically to dilate even the smallest capillaries which helps relieve headache and migraine pain.

Quercetin is a bioflavonoid, a type of plant pigment found in herbs and plants. It is an antioxidant that has been found to block destructive structural changes in cells, which helps to prevent abnormal cell growth. It also inhibits the synthesis of enzymes that can cause allergic reactions. Quercetin prevents migraine attacks especially those triggered by food allergies. Recommended doses are 125 to 250 mg, 3 times daily between meals. Ginkgo has few side effects and when use with SSRIs it has been reported to reverse the sexual dysfunction side effects caused by SSRIs [72, 73].

Other teas reported to relieve headaches include: **ginger tea**, which is believed to relax blood vessels in the head, acts as a natural opiate in the brain that relieves pain, and reduces prostaglandins, **chamomile, lemon balm,** and **linden** (flowers of the lime tree) all are believed to act as sedatives to the nervous system. Researchers believe linden can aid in healing migraines and tension headaches by improving blood circulation.

Lavender, a herb with sedative properties is used as an essential oil in tincture and has been used to treat muscle spasms, nervousness, and headaches for over 200 years in Europe. A 1994 study on headaches used the essential oils of **peppermint** and **eucalyptus** and found they relaxed both mind and muscles. When those herbs were diluted in alcohol, then sponged on the foreheads of study participants, both reduced sensitivity to headaches. The essentials oils of peppermint, eucalyptus, and lavender can also be used to make a compress that can be used on the forehead or back of the neck to relieve headache pain. A German study reported that peppermint oil with ethyl alcohol was most effective in relieving headache pain when dabbed on the forehead [74, 75].

Aromatherapy

Aromatherapy uses **essential oils** (highly concentrated solutions from plants) to heal a variety of disorders and illnesses. Essential oils are used in cosmetics, perfumes, soaps, bath oils, massage oils, inhalations, and internally. A number of essential oils are used in aromatherapy to relieve headaches and migraines. Chamomile, lavender, and marjoram essential oils have anti-inflammatory, antispasmodic, sedative anticonvulsive and antidepressant properties that relieves headaches and migraines. Mint essential oils such as pennyroyal, peppermint, and spearmint, and rosemary and rose essential oil have stimulating properties that help relieve headaches and migraines.

Therapy can be increased by combining a number of essential oils for use in diffusers (inhalation) or in a massage oil. For headaches chamomile, peppermint, rosewood, spearmint, and lavender can be combined. A blend of lavender, marjoram, melissa, peppermint, and spearmint are recommended for migraines [76, 77].

Medical Devices

Biofeedback training has been successful in treating chronic headaches and migraines. Biofeedback training can instruct headache suffers on how to control certain involuntary functions of the body, such as heart rate or body temperature, which can, in turn, ward off headaches. Biofeedback training can help stabilize or alter blood vessels in the head that narrow and constrict during migraines and tension headaches. By raising the temperature of a part of the body, such as the hands, blood flow is redirected from the head relieving pressure in cranial blood vessels.

Electrically stimulated biofeedback has also shown to be effect in treating migraines. **Transcutaneous Electrical Stimulation** (TENS) involves the production and transmission of electrical energy from the surface of the skin to the nervous system. The rationale behind this therapy is the process by which the small, uncovered pain fibers can be controlled by the larger covered fibers, thus reducing pain. The control of these fibers would manage pain symptoms. For headaches the TENS instrument, a small stimulator, is connected to electrodes placed on the skin's surface, usually over the site of the pain. The patient can control the amount of stimulation for a specified interval, about five to ten minutes. TENS has been shown to be effective in a placebo-controlled trial in the treatment of patients migraine and tension headaches. In the study 55 percent showed improvement with TENS, compared to 18 percent in the placebo group [78, 79, 80, 81].

A nerve stimulation procedure has shown to be highly effective in reducing the severity of cluster headaches. A study reports that a procedure involving positioning a fine electrode under the skin in the base of the skull that is attached to a pacemaker-like device elsewhere in the body. The electrode stimulates the occipital nerve relieving the intense burning and stabbing pain located behind the eye of the cluster headache sufferer. This procedure has been effective for chronic cluster headache patients that have not responded to other treatments [82].

Another device called the **Transcranial Magnetic Stimulation** device (TMS) is waiting FDA approval for use with migraines. The TMS transmits magnetic pulses that interrupt the "hyperexcitability" of neurons in the brain, that many experts believe is to blame for launching the migraine. The TMS device is a small portable device weighing about 3 pounds. Patients grasp the box's two handles holding it to their heads when they feel the aura of a migraine coming on. The magnetic pulses have been found to greatly reduce the pain associated with the migraine within two hours of using the device [83].

Acupuncture

Acupuncture, the Chinese art of manipulating energy channels in the body, has been shown to relieve headaches and migraines. These energy channels, or meridians are blocked by needles thus blocking the headache pain. A study from New Zealand using acupuncture showed that as few as 12 acupuncture treatments resulted in fewer and less severe migraine attacks. Another study found that acupuncture reduced the severity and frequency of migraines in 40 percent of the individuals in the study by 40 to 100 percent. Acupuncture may work by normalization of serotonin levels, and there are no significant adverse effects using this treatment [84, 85, 86].

Exercise

Exercise may not be a cure for headaches or migraines, but it doses strengthen overall health and help relieve stress that can contribute to the problem. Stress can cause negative changes in the body, including blood vessel constriction, muscle tension, and the release of stress chemicals, like adrenaline and catecholamines, into the blood stream, which can increase the potential for migraines. Relaxation is the antithesis of stress, widening the blood vessels, decreasing muscle tension, and dissipating excess stress chemicals.

Exercise increases circulation bringing more oxygen to the tissues, clearing away toxins faster. Lack of oxygen and toxic buildup are two instigators of migraines. There is evidence migraine sufferers produce lower amounts of endorphins, the body's natural painkiller, than those who don't get migraines. Those who exercise regularly tend to have higher overall energy levels and a greater resistance to fatigue, a common trigger to headaches and migraines. Regular exercise increases high quality of deep sleep, improves digestion, helps strengthen the excretory system, removing wastes and toxins from the body, all helping to alleviate headaches and migraines [87].

Dental Appliance

A study by Dr. Phillip Lamey from Royal Hospital in Northern Ireland found that by having migraine sufferers wear a dental appliance (like a sports mouth guard) their migraine attacks dropped by 60 percent. The appliance kept migraine sufferer's teeth from grinding while asleep, greatly reducing the incidence of migraine attacks. It was most effect for individuals that experienced migraines in the morning or those that have at least two attacks per week. He reported after a year of wearing the appliance, 70 percent of the patients had their migraine attacks cease completely [88].

Migraines May Decrease with Age

A 12 year Swedish study, from 1994 to 2006, of 364 migraine patients (200 women, 174 men) of an average age of 55, found that migraine attacks diminish. The study found that the average duration of migraine attacks is 25 years. They reported that 80 percent of the people in the study had fewer migraines, with less pain, lasting of shorter duration. The study concludes that for most people, migraines are not a progressive disease [89].

CONCLUSIONS:

The pain from a headache can range from a mild throbbing to a debilitating migraine. It is estimated that 80 million Americans experience headaches, 50 million have experienced a migraine, and 28 million suffer from migraines continually. The economic cost of migraines is enormous, with 150 million lost days from work or school in the U.S. and $13 million in lost productivity per year. Women are more likely than men to suffer from migraines, as 70 percent of migraine patients are female. Thirty percent of migraine suffers have their first attack before age ten, and the disorder is very prevalent among adolescents and young adults. Over $20 billion a year is spent by suffers desperate for relief from headaches and migraines.

Migraine incidence appears to be increasing at a rate of 56 percent in women and 34 percent in men between 1980 and 1990, possibly from more stress on the workforce. The most common types of headaches are tension headaches and migraines. Stress, irregular sleep, hormonal shifts, depression, eyestrain, and food allergies are the most common causes. And, just as in other mental disorders there is a variety of treatment options based on the cause and severity of the disorder.

Headaches are usually divided into four categories; tension headaches, organic headaches, and vascular headaches that can be either cluster headaches or migraines. Tension headaches (or muscle contraction headaches) are believed to be caused by muscle tension. Some 75 to 80 percent of the headaches people get fall into this category. And, 90 percent of the population gets this type of headache from time to time. Pain is usually felt in the back of the head and neck. The pain may envelop the whole head, and feel like the head is in a vise. People with these headaches often have sore shoulders and a sore neck as well, and tension headaches may last for days without relief, except for during sleep. Tension headaches usually begin during adult life, however, 10 to 20 percent of people report getting this type of headache as children and teenagers. Men and women get this type of headache about equally. Tension headaches can be categorized as episodic tension-type headaches (ETTH) or chronic tension-type headaches (CTTH). The prevalence rate of ETTH was 38.3 percent, with the rate peaking in 30 to 39 year-olds of 42.3 percent in males and 46.9 percent in women.

Organic headaches are usually a symptom of another ailment. It could be a sign of inflammation around the brain, elevated blood pressure, a buildup of fluid around the brain, or even a brain tumor. Less than one percent of the headaches are organic, but the underlying problems may be life threatening.

Vascular headaches gain their name from the process by which blood vessels in the head expand or dilate, and cause the pain of cluster headaches or migraine attacks. Cluster headaches usually affect one side of the head, with severe pain around the eye. It may radiate from above the affected eye to the temple and to the jaw or gums on the same side or more rarely over half of the head. The cluster headache often occurs in bouts, with each lasting from four to eight weeks. The attack builds within a few minutes and lasts for a total of about 45 minutes. Several attacks may occur each day during the cluster period and may even wake the suffer from sleep. Cluster headaches appear more often in men (90 percent) than women, typically starts in their 30's, and are rare, affecting fewer than one percent of the population.

Migraines are classified into classic migraines (with aura) and common migraines (without aura). Up to 70 percent of migraine suffers have both types of migraines. Classic migraine constitutes only about 35 percent of all migraine attacks. The headache, nausea, and vomiting of this migraine attack are preceded by flashing lights or other sensory symptoms. A suffer may complain about bright stars that pass across the field of vision and even a temporary loss of sight, or double vision occurs. There may also be a tingling and pins and needles sensation in one hand or arm, or around the mouth. The migraine with aura usually has four stages; the prodrome stage, where symptoms start, which may include feeling tired, stiff neck, thirst, sensitivity to light and sound, irritability, and craving for sweets. The aura stage, characterized by seeing lights, tingling sensations and photosensitivity, the third stage is where the headache occurs, which is usually one-sided in the forehead or temples, and the final stage or recovery stage, where the pain subsides.

Common migraines, differ from classic migraines where the individual does not experience the aura. Sixty-five percent of people who suffer from migraines experience this kind of migraine. It progresses in three stages, with the same symptoms; the prodrome, the headache, and the recovery stage.

Headaches and migraines have a variety of causes and treatment should be related to the cause. The brain itself does not feel pain. Headache pain has its source in the nerves located in the muscles and blood vessels of the face, neck and scalp, in the nerves running between the back of the brain, and in the brain's blood vessels. Ten percent of headaches may be caused by organic sources such as brain tumors, hemorrhaging into the layers of the meninges or the brain, aneurysms, meningitis, temporal arteritis, or head injuries. It may be caused by obstructive sleep apnea, TMJ or eye strain.

Acute tension headaches can be caused by stressful events, chronic tension headaches are frequent, at least twice a week, and may be caused by stress, and associated with depression and sleep disturbance. Chronic tension headaches may also be caused by arthritis, neck injuries, spinal tumors, or congenital deformities. Sinus headaches are caused by inflammation of the sinus cavities.

Migraines are estimated to affect 8 to 10 percent of all men and 18 to 20 percent of all women at some point in their lives. The disorder affects more women then men (up to 75 percent are women), and the onset of migraines break down to 25 percent getting their first migraine by age ten, 56 percent by age 13, 75 percent by age 30, and 90 percent by age 40. Migraines are known as vascular headaches because they involve the blood vessels in the face, head and neck. Sometimes they become unnaturally narrowed (constricted) other times they become abnormally widened (dilated). If the blood vessels in the head are constricted there is an accumulation of chemical irritants within the blood vessels, since a normal flow of blood is not pulsing through to wash the irritants away. The vasoconstriction seems to set off the opposite reaction, vasodilatation in the blood vessels on the surface of the brain and scalp. This corresponds to the throbbing, painful stage of the migraine, that seems as though the head might burst from an excess of blood.

Theories as to what sets off this process of vasoconstriction and vasodilatation include changes in levels of serotonin, that effects amines like noradrenaline, histamine, and dopamine, and eating foods that are high in certain amines (such as chocolate, cheese and alcohol). This sensitivity to amines are often found in migraine suffers to where they seemingly have lower defenses to these chemicals found in foods. An over-sensitivity that may cause a migraine is an individual's over reaction to stress which produces adrenaline, which in turn can cause a headache.

Another factor that is believed to be responsible for half of all migraines are related to magnesium levels in the body. Magnesium helps to regulate serotonin levels in the brain, and it has been found that migraine suffers lack this essential mineral. Without magnesium, serotonin levels are not properly regulated, blood vessels do not retain their proper size, inflammation sets in, and a migraine develops. Magnesium also helps other chemicals in the body that regulate dilation and constriction.

Other theories as to the cause of migraines involves an oversensitive hypothalamus gland, hypoglycemia (overactive pancreas that produces too much insulin) that stimulates the adrenal glands to produce catecholamines that constrict the blood vessels. The catecholamines trigger the production of prostaglandins that dilate blood vessels which produces the throbbing pain of a migraine. In addition to the effects of sugar causing migraines in hypoglycemics, many people have specific food allergies that have been shown to cause headaches and migraines. These food triggers include: pork; game and organ meats; smoked and cured, aged and packaged meat; herring, caviar, and smoked fish; vinegar; pickled and fermented foods; aged cheese; products high in yeasts and tyramines; chocolate; sugar and all products made with processed sugar or corn syrup; yogurt; the pods of lima beans, navy beans, and peas; flavor enhancers such as MSG; caffeine; and alcoholic beverages, especially red wine.

Studies on food allergies related to the cause of migraine range from 30 to 93 percent responsible for the migraine.

Nicotine in tobacco is a vasoconstrictor that the body becomes dependent on. As the body needs ever higher amounts to keep the blood vessels constricted rebound effects occur leading to headaches. In addition smokers have large amounts of carbon monoxide and carboxyhemoglobin in their blood, substances that displace oxygen and cause a lack of oxygen in the brain. Lack of oxygen causes blood vessels to dilate in an attempt to carry more blood to the brain, which may trigger a headache.

Environmental triggers can cause migraines, the most common being related to allergy toxins such as pollen, dust (dust mites), pets (especially cats), gas stove emissions, household cleaners, perfume, cosmetics, fabric cleaners, hairspray, air fresheners, cigarette smoke, car exhausts, smog, pesticides, and natural gas. Changes in the weather can increase the frequency and severity of migraines. Springtime encourages migraines because of the proliferation of allergens in the air. The heat and humidity of summer encourages mold growth, the release of grass pollens, and the proliferation of heavy smog. Rainstorms causes a drop in barometric pressure that changes the ratio of positive to negative ions in the air, and an increase in the positive ions carries with them more allergens that attach themselves to the positive ions. Inadequate sleep or poor quality REM sleep can cause a migraine as well.

Prescription medications can cause migraines such as agents used for treating high blood pressure, medications for treating heart disease, and arthritis, and estrogen used in birth control pills and hormonal replacement therapy cause migraines in some women. Migraines are believed to have genetic links. About 70 percent of migraine sufferers have a family history of migraines. The incidence of migraines is especially high if both parents have suffered from migraines.

There are several treatment options for headaches and migraines depending on the severity and frequency of the pain and the effort the individual wants to place in uncovering the cause. For tension and migraine headaches that occur once a week or less, OTC pain relievers can be effective such as aspirin, acetaminophen, a combination of aspirin or acetaminophen and caffeine, and nonsteroidal anti-inflammatory drugs, such as ibuprofen and naproxen sodium. If these medications fail to produce results, prescription painkillers may work such as *abortive drugs* to stop migraines in progress, and *prophylactic drugs* to prevent future ones from striking. Abortive drugs include corticosteroids, ergot derivatives, opioids/narcotics, NASAIDS, triptans, and combination drugs. Prophylactic drugs include antidepressants, SSRIs, antiseizure medications, beta-blockers, calcium channel blockers, MAO inhibitors, and botox. All of these medications carry warnings of possible side effects of stomach ulcers, chest tightness, weight gain or loss, nausea, diarrhea or constipation, high blood pressure, irritability, anxiety, depression, insomnia, blurred vision, hair loss, sexual dysfunction, addiction, and dangerous interactions with other drugs. Overuse of both prescription medications and over-the-counter painkillers can lead to drug rebound headaches. When this happens, a once-effective drug no longer produces results, and when the dose wears off, another, worse headache appears.

Naturopathic therapy for headaches and migraines uses nutritional interventions, herbal remedies, aromatherapy and physical therapies such as biofeedback training, acupuncture, exercise, dental aids and electrical or magnetic stimulation devices. There are very few side effects reported with these therapies unless the individual uses more than the recommended amounts for the treatment or uses it in conjunction with prescription medications that may have amplifying effects.

Naturopathic treatment for headaches and migraines tries to uncover the cause first. Dietary and nutritional evaluations are conducted to determine if allergies, toxins, or nutritional deficiencies are the cause of the headaches or migraines. If so, that toxin or food is eliminated. Vitamin and mineral deficiencies include the B vitamins: riboflavin (B2), niacin (B3), pantothenic acid (B5), pyridoxine (B6), and cobalamin (B12), that helps the body cope with stress, aids in intermediary metabolism, and the metabolism of sugar and carbohydrates. Niacin, due to its vasodilatory effects, has long been recommended in the popular literature for treatment of migraine headaches. B vitamins are depleted by caffeine, birth control pills, alcohol, and stress. Vitamin A heals the mucous membranes, vitamin C, with bioflavonoids constricts and cleans veins, and vitamin E increases oxygen in the blood.

Minerals such as potassium, iron, iodine, and zinc are essential for proper nervous system functioning. Essential fatty acids (EFAs) may help reduce the frequency of headaches. EPA, an omega-3 fatty acid, directs the cascade of chemical alterations that lead from the raw fatty acid to the final prostaglandin products toward the production of good prostaglandins by blocking the step that produces arachidonic acid, the forerunner of all the "bad" messengers. To increase this production of good prostaglandins there must be a balance between two EFAs, linoleic acid (GLA) found in products like evening primrose oil and EPA found in cold water fish. The ratio of GLA and EPA is recommended at 1:4.

Feverfew is believed to be effective in treatment of migraines due to parthenolide, a substance in the herb that helps dampen the inflammation process associated with migraines. It may also mitigate the effects of histamine and arachidonic acid that contributes to headaches and their symptoms. Feverfew is also believed to inhibit the secretion of serotonin from platelets, decrease blood vessel response to vasconstrictors, and it inhibits the production of inflammatory biochemicals. Side effects of feverfew are few and very mild and the herb is considered nontoxic.

Other nutritional therapies that have been studied in migraine treatment include the use of cayenne pepper, and quercetin. Cayenne pepper contains the active ingredient capsaicin, that acts as a potent inhibitor of platelet aggregation and thereby relieves pain. Quercetin is a bioflavonoid that helps to promote cell health and inhibits many of the pathways of inflammation. It is also believe to act as protection against foods that may induce migraine attacks.

Herbal therapy treatment of headaches and migraines use calming, regulating and restoring herbs. Tension-headache sufferers can benefit from herbs that soothe the body and mind. Teas made from chamomile or passionflower help relax stiff muscles in the head and neck, reducing pressure on the blood vessels. Valerian has been used for centuries in folk medicine to treat headaches and migraines. Ephedra, or ma-huang, a Chinese herb, has been used in traditional Chinese medicine for over 2,000 years to treat headache. Skullcap is a member of the mint family and has been found to be a nerve tonic and sedative for relieving anxiety, neuralgia, insomnia and headaches. Willow bark is considered a natural aspirin. For more than 2,000 years people in the northern hemisphere used willow bark as a wash for external ulcers, and internally to reduce fevers, relieve aches, pains, rheumatism, arthritis, and headaches. Thyme is commonly used as a culinary herb, but it has also been used to treat tension headaches when used in a tea. Doug quai is used to prevent migraine attacks by blocking the production of prostaglandins and has anti-inflammatory properties. Ginkgo is believed to help migraines by enhancing cerebral circulation.

Other teas reported to relieve headaches include: ginger tea, chamomile, lemon balm, and linden. All are believed to act as sedatives to the nervous system. Lavender, a herb with sedative properties is used as an essential oil in tincture and has been used to treat muscle spasms, nervousness, and headaches for over 200 years in Europe. The essential oils of peppermint and eucalyptus relax both mind and muscles, and when diluted in alcohol and sponged on the foreheads they reduced the sensitivity to headaches.

Aromatherapy has been found to reduce headaches and migraines by using essential oils in bath oils, massage oils, inhalations, and internally. Chamomile, lavender, and marjoram essential oils have anti-inflammatory, antispasmodic, sedative anticonvulsive and antidepressant properties that relieves headaches and migraines. Mint essential oils such as pennyroyal, peppermint, and spearmint, and rosemary and rose essential oil have stimulating properties that help relieve headaches and migraines.

Other therapies that have been found to reduce the frequency or relieve headaches and migraines include biofeedback training, acupuncture, exercise, a dental appliance , and new electrically or magnetically stimulation devices.

Holistic Mental Health for Headaches & Migraines Specific Recommendations:

Treatment for headaches and migraines should be based on the frequency and severity of them. For an occasional headache or migraine (less than one per month) OTC medication may be adequate. Prescription medications may also be effective for short-term treatment, if no serious side effects are encountered. However, medications do not uncover the cause of the problem. For frequent headaches and migraines treatment should begin by determining the cause. The most common origin of headaches and migraines are food allergies. Determining if there is an allergen or toxin, by carefully analyzing the diet and possible environmental toxins exposed to, and eliminating exposure to that food or toxin may be all the treatment that is necessary.

If a specific allergy can not be determined the following steps should be taken:

- Follow a natural diet of fresh vegetable and fruits, whole-wheat products with protein from cold water fish or turkey. Eliminate processed foods, foods high in sugar, and foods that contain additives.

- Eliminate caffeine and nicotine.

- Take a multi-vitamin/mineral daily with extra B-complex (1 in a.m. and 1 in p.m.), vitamin C (2-3,000 mg per day, take in two doses), vitamin E (200 to 400 IUs, per day), calcium, magnesium and zinc (can be taken in 1 supplement, take 1,200 to 1,500 mg of calcium, 300 to 400 mg of magnesium, and 20 to 30 mg of zinc in 2 doses per day).

- Add feverfew daily of 50 mg in the a.m. and 50 mg in p.m. Increase during headache or migraine attacks to 500 to 1,000 mg.

- Unless cold water fish is eaten daily take EFA supplements (500 mg of evening primrose oil, and 1,000 mg of EPA fish oil daily).

- Rather than coffee drink decaffeinated chamomile, passionflower, ginger, lemon balm, linden, mint, or peppermint tea daily.

- Take a hot bath or get a therapeutic massage with essential oils of lavender, chamomile, peppermint, rosewood, spearmint, marjoram, or Melissa.

- Make sure you are getting adequate sleep. Use relaxation techniques in order to get 7 or 8 hours of restful sleep.

- If feverfew does not appear to be effective after two months of daily supplements try willow bark, skullcap, doug quai or ginkgo supplements.

- If sufficient pain relief is not obtained from the above recommendations, go to an acupuncturist or try a clinic that specializes in biofeedback training.

- The above treatment proceeds from the least harmful of side effects, therefore, the "last resort" of pain relief should be prescription pain relievers, and are recommended for only temporary use only.

Treatment for medical conditions should always be conducted by your healthcare professional. According to the FDA only physicians are allowed to prescribe medications, and the suggestions in this book are for dietary changes and/or supplements only.

"The hardest thing in life is to learn which bridge
to burn and which bridge to cross."
~ Laurence J. Peter

CHAPTER VII:
OTHER MENTAL DISORDERS:
Bipolar Disorder, Schizophrenia,

Bipolar Disorder

Bipolar Disorder or previously termed *manic-depressive* disorder is classified as a mood disorder. Mood disorders have been observed as far back as recorded history allows. The term *melancholia* is credited to Hippocrates. Descriptions of bipolar disorder date back to the 2nd century where Aretaes of Cappadocia reported an association between melancholia and mania. By the end of the 18th century another important contribution was made in understanding mood disorders by Krapelin. In 1896 he separated functional psychoses into two groups: dementia praecox and manic-depressive psychosis.

In 1917, Freud published *Mourning and Melancholia,* that described his theories of depression. In it he stated that depression and grief had in common the process of mourning. He further observed that although grief is a healthy response, it differed from melancholia in that melancholia involves ambivalent and intense hostile feelings formerly associated with the object. The theories of the origins of mood disorders, and the controversy the continues today, can be credited to Krapelin (biological basis) and Freud (environmental reactions)[1].

The prevalence of major depression in one's lifetime can be as high as 18 percent. However, bipolar disorder affects only one percent of the population. Woman are at a greater risk for depression, with the age of onset in the late 20's, but bipolar disorder is equal among women and men with the average

age of onset in the early 20's. According to the National Institute of Mental Health, about 5.7 million American adults have bipolar disorder [2].

A new study suggests that children born from older fathers are at an increased risk of developing bipolar disorder. In the September, 2008 issue of *Archives of Psychiatry* a study found that children born to fathers in their mid-50s and older had a 37 percent higher risk for bipolar disorder than children born to fathers in their early 20s. Researchers believe the cause of this could be in genetic mutations in the sperm of the older fathers [3].

Genetic Links

The largest study to date has shown that Bipolar Disorder and Schizophrenia may share a common genetic cause. A study from Sweden involving 9 million Swedes from 2 million families, reviewing data from 3 decades revealed a number of similarities between the two disorders. In the study 40,500 people with bipolar disorder, and 36,000 people with schizophrenia were identified.

The study found first degree relatives such as parents, siblings, or offspring of people with either bipolar disorder or schizophrenia were at an increased risk for both of these conditions. If a sibling had schizophrenia, full siblings were 9 times more likely to have schizophrenia and 4 times more likely to have bipolar disorder. If a sibling had bipolar disorder, they were 8 times more likely to have bipolar disorder and 4 times more likely to have schizophrenia. Half siblings who shared the same mother were 3.6 times more likely to have schizophrenia if their half sibling had schizophrenia, and 4.5 times more likely to have bipolar disorder if their half sibling had bipolar disorder. Half siblings that shared the same father had a 2.7-fold increase in schizophrenia risk, and a 2.4-fold increase in bipolar disorder [4].

Classification of Bipolar Disorder

Bipolar Disorder is classified as a Mood Disorder in the *DSM-IV-TR*. Other Mood Disorders in this classification includes Major Depressive Disorder and Dysthymic Disorder (see Chapter IV). Bipolar Disorder is further classified as ***Bipolar I Disorder:*** characterized by one or more Manic or mixed episodes, usually accompanied by Major Depressive Episodes. And, ***Bipolar II Disorder:*** characterized by one or more Major Depressive Episodes accompanied by a least one Hypomanic Episode [5].

Criteria for Manic Episode[6]:

A. A distinct period of abnormally and persistently elevated, expansive, or irritable mood, lasting at least 1 week (or any duration if hospitalization is necessary).

B. During the period of mood disturbance, three (or more) of the following symptoms have persisted (for if the mood is only irritable) and have been present to a significant degree:

1. Inflated self-esteem or grandiosity.
2. Decreased need for sleep (e.g., feels rested after only 3 hours of sleep).
3. More talkative than usual or pressure to keep talking.
4. Flight of ideas or subjective experience that thoughts are racing.
5. Distractibility (I.e., attention too easily drawn to unimportant or irrelevant external stimuli).
6. Increase in goal-directed activity (either socially, at work or school, or sexually) or psychomotor agitation.
7. Excessive involvement in pleasurable activities that have a high potential for painful consequences (e.g., engaging in unrestrained buying sprees, sexual indiscretions, or foolish business investments).

C. The symptoms do not meet the criteria for a Mixed Episode.

D. The mood disturbance is sufficiently severe to cause marked impairment in occupational functioning or in usual social activities or relationships with others, or to necessitate hospitalization to prevent harm to self or others, or there are psychotic features.

E. The symptoms are not due to the direct physiological effects of a substance (e.g., a drug of abuse, a medication, or other treatment) or a general medical condition (e.g., hyperthyroidism).

A Mixed Episode is characterized by a period of time (lasting at least 1 week) in which the criteria are met both for a Manic Episode and for a Major Depressive Episode nearly every day. The Individual experiences rapidly alternating moods (sadness, irritability, euphoria) accompanied by symptoms of a Manic Episode and a Major Depressive Episode. Symptoms include agitation, insomnia, appetite dysregulation, psychotic features, and suicidal thinking. The disturbance must be severe enough to cause marked impairment in social or occupational functioning, or to require hospitalization, or it is characterized by psychotic features. The disturbance is not due to the direct physiological effects of a substance (e.g. drugs of abuse, a medication, or other treatment) or a general medical condition (e.g., hyperthyroidism) [7].

A bipolar disorder **Hypomanic Episode** is defined where there is a distinct period of abnormal and persistently elevated, expansive, or irritable mood that lasts at least 4 days. This period of abnormal mood must also be accompanied by at least three additional symptoms such as; inflated self-esteem, or grandiosity (not delusional), decreased need for sleep, pressure of speech, flight of ideas, distractibility, increased involvement in goal-directed activities or psychomotor agitation, and excessive involvement in pleasurable activities that have a high consequence for painful consequences. If the mood is irritable rather than elevated or expansive, at least four of the above symptoms must be present.

The elevated mood in a Hypomanic Episode is usually euphoric, cheerful, or high. Although the person's mood may be infectious, but it is recognized as uncharacteristic by those that know the individual. The may also alternate between euphoria and irritability. Inflated self-esteem and uncritical self-confidence is present rather than marked grandiosity. There is often a decreased need for sleep and increased energy. The speech of a person in a Hypomanic Episode can be somewhat louder and more rapid than usual, but is not typically difficult to interrupt [8].

When the criteria is met for Manic, Mixed or Hypomanic Episodes and the criteria for a Major Depressive Disorder the diagnosis becomes Bipolar Disorder:

Symptoms/ Criteria for Major Depressive Episode[9]:

Five (or more) of the following symptoms have been present during the same two week period and represent a change from previous functioning; at least one of the symptoms is either depressed mood or lost of interest in pleasure:

- Depressed mood most of the day, nearly every day, as indicated by either subjective report or observation made by others.

- Markedly diminished interest in pleasure in all, or almost all, activities most of the day, nearly every day.

- Significant weight loss when not dieting or weight gain (change of more than 5% of body weight in a month) or decrease or increase in appetite nearly every day.

- Insomnia or hypersomnia nearly every day.

- Psychomotor agitation or retardation nearly every day.

- Fatigue or loss of energy nearly every day.

- Feelings of worthlessness or excessive or inappropriate guilt (which may be delusional) nearly every day.

- Diminished ability to think or concentrate, or indecisiveness, nearly every day

- Recurrent thoughts of death, recurrent suicidal ideation without a specific plan, or a suicide attempt or a specific plan for committing suicide.

- The symptoms do not meet the criteria for a Mixed Episode.

- The symptoms cause clinically significant distress or impairment in social, occupational, or other important areas of functioning.

- The symptoms are not due to the direct physiological effects of a substance or a general medical condition.

- The symptoms are not better accounted for bereavement, i.e., after the loss of a loved one, the symptoms persist for longer than 2 months or are characterized by marked functional impairment, morbid preoccupation with worthlessness, suicidal ideation, psychotic symptoms, or psychomotor retardation.

Allopathic Treatment for Bipolar Disorder:

Table 7-1
*Summary of Allopathic Treatment for
Bipolar Disorder* [10-14]:

Drug: (brand name)	**Acting mechanism:**	**Possible side effects:**
Lithium, lithium-carbonate: (*Eskalith, Eskalith CR, Carbolith, Cibalith-S, Duralith, Lithane, Lithizine, Lithobid, Lithonate, Lithotabs*)	Helps correct chemical imbalance in the brain's transmission of nerve impulses that influence mood and behavior.	Frequent urination, hand tremor, mild thirst, nausea, abdominal pain, blackouts, confusion, dehydration, dizziness, dry hair or hair loss, dry mouth, fatigue, hallucinations, increased salivation, indigestion, involuntary tongue movements, involuntary urination, irregular heartbeat, loss of appetite, low blood pressure, muscle rigidity or twitching, painful joints, poor memory, seizures, sexual dysfunction, slurred speech, vision problems, vomiting, weakness, weight gain or loss, coma.

Antipsychotics: **Areipiprazole** *(Abilify)*, **Clozapine** *(Clorazil)*, **Olanzapine** *(Symbyax, Zyprexa)*, **Quatrain** *(Seroquel)*, **Risperidone** *(Risperdal)*, **Ziprasidone** *(Geodon)*	It appears to alleviate symptoms of mania by blocking certain nerve impulses between nerve cells.	Abdominal pain, abnormal gait, agitation, anxiety, back pain, behavior problems, blood in urine, blurred vision, chest pain, constipation, dehydration, dizziness, drowsiness, dry mouth, skin or eyes, extreme low or high blood pressure, fever, headache, insomnia, joint pain, involuntary movements, muscle rigidity, nausea, nervousness, tremors, weight gain, sexual dysfunction, stroke, heart attack.
Anticonvulsants: **Carbamazepine** *(Tegretol)*, **Lamotrigine** *(Lamictal)*, **Oxcarbazepine** *Trileptal)* **Valproic acid, Divalproex -sodium,** *(Depakote, Myproic Acid)*,	Increases concentration of gamma amino butyric acid, which inhibits nerve transmission in parts of the brain.	Abdominal pain, abnormal thinking, breathing difficulty, bronchitis, constipation, depression, diarrhea, dizziness, drowsiness, fever, flu symptoms, hair loss, headache, insomnia, involuntary movements, muscle or joint pain, nausea, weakness, nervousness, tremors, weight loss or gain, sexual dysfunction, high blood pressure, liver damage.
Benzodiazepines: **Alprazolam** *(Xanax)*, **Clonazepam** *(Klonopin)*, **Diazepam** *(Valium)*, **Lorazepam** *(Ativan)*	Reduces excitability of nerve fibers in the brain, thus inhibiting the repetitive spread of nerve impulses. Produces calmness.	Dizziness, drowsiness, unsteadiness, fatigue, involuntary movements, blurred vision, confusion, memory loss, lightheadedness. May be habit forming and addictive.

Naturopathic Therapy for Bipolar Disorder:

Bipolar Disorder can be treated holistically by addressing symptoms of the mania and the depression. However, due to the severity of symptoms an individual may experience with Bipolar Disorder therapy should be prescribed by a naturopathic physician.

To reduce the symptoms of mania, calming herbs such as:

American ginseng, *Panax quinquefolius:*

American ginseng is a cooling, sedating "yin" tonic that helps bring balance and harmony to the body. It used to reduce stress and anxiety, and calm the body. Ginseng's medicinal properties are concentrated its thick, fleshy root that resembles a white or yellow carrot [15].

Kava kava, *Piper methysticum:*

Researchers first began looking into the relaxant properties of kava in the 1950's and recent clinical studies have supported its use in treating anxiety and stress. Kava appears to work by modifying rather than blocking brain chemicals that affect emotions. This is unlike prescription anti-anxiety drugs that produce a calming effect by blocking these neurochemicals. However, when these neurochemicals are blocked by medications other senses are dulled especially mental alertness. Kava elevates mood and increases mental alertness [16].

Lavender, *Lavandula officinalis:*

Lavender is considered an aromatic healing herb. Therapeutic properties of lavender are used in relieving stress and anxiety, tension, insomnia, headache and nausea. Taken internally lavender is available as teas, dried flowers, powdered herb, capsules and tinctures. Externally, the essential oil of lavender is used in aromatherapy to promote relaxation, stimulate the mind clarify thinking, encourage creativity, and relieve depression [17].

Skullcap/Virginian, *Scutellaria lateniflora:*

Skullcap has been used as a remedy for sleep disorders and as a tranquilizer. The leaves and blue flowers of the Virginian species of skullcap have long been used in many herbal sleep remedies and tranquilizing teas. Native Americans regularly used skullcap as a sedative and indigestion treatment. Some holistic practitioners believe that skullcap is particularly effective in neutralizing negative emotions, like anger, and is helpful in enhancing the meditative state.

Skullcap is available as a dried herb, tea, tincture, and capsules. Side effects of skullcap could include upset stomachs, diarrhea, twitching, convulsions or drowsiness if too much is taken [18].

Valerian, Valeriana officinalis:

Valerian is often thought of as the "valium" of the plant kingdom. It has been used for over the 1,000 years as a relaxant. Recent research has confirmed valerian as a mild and safe tranquilizer that is particularly useful for treating anxiety, nervous tension, stress and panic attacks. Valerian is also reported as a good treatment as a sleep aid where, unlike pharmaceutical sedatives it does not interfere with dream states or rapid eye movement.

Valerian is taken internally for anxiety, nervousness, and tension, stress related headache, muscle ache, and internal pains, menstrual cramps, and insomnia. It is available as a dried herb, capsules, tincture, and teas, alone or in combination with other calming herbs such as St. John's wort, passionflower or Kava kava. Recommended dosage in *Valepotriate* tablets is 50 mg, 3 times a day. Over-consumption of the herb may lead to headache, restlessness, nausea, drowsiness or blurred vision. It should not be used when on prescription tranquilizers or sedatives due to additive effect [19].

Passionflower, Passiflora incarnata:

Passion flower was introduced to Europe in the late 1800's for its calming effect on the central nervous system. The flower, vine and leaves of this herb contain alkaloids and flavonoids that, in laboratory studies, have demonstrated sedating effects. Herbalist recommend it as a sedative, digestive aid or pain reliever. Passionflower also reduces high blood pressure. It is most used for chronic stress relief, anxiety and insomnia. Because it dilates blood vessels it is being tested as a heart disease preventive.

Passionflower used as dried or fresh leaves, capsules, tea or tincture. For anxiety 1 dropper of tincture in warm water four times a day is recommended. Passionflower should not be used with other prescription sedatives as over medication can occur, and pregnant women should not use it as it may stimulate uterine muscles. Mild side effects of upset stomach, nausea, vomiting, diarrhea, and sleepiness may occur with overuse [20].

Chamomile, *Matricaria chamomilla:*

Researchers believe elements in the oil of the flowers, primarily apigenin and azulene are responsible for calming the central nervous system, relax the digestive track, speed healing and fight infection. Chamomile is also rich in calcium, magnesium, and iron. The warm tea is calming and helps induce relaxation and promote sleep. Soaking in a chamomile bath will not only calm nerves it will also relieve minor aches and pains. Taken internally, as in teas chamomile has sedating properties, antispasmodic, pain-relieving and wound-healing properties.

Chamomile is used as dried or fresh flowers, tea, tincture, and essential oil. It is often combined with other herbs for relaxation and sleep such as Kava kava, valerian and passionflower. People who have ragweed allergies may also have allergic reactions to chamomile other adverse side effects have not been reported [21].

Lemon balm, *Melissa officinalis:*

Lemon balm, is a close relative to chamomile. It is the mildest of the sedating herbs and is often prescribed for children. It is especially effective in relaxing the body and calming the emotions prior to sleep. Therapeutically lemon balm has antispasmodic action, is mildly sedating, and relieves indigestion.

Lemon balm's sedating action seems to specifically to target brain activity, and is frequently prescribed for insomnia, or other sleep problems in which there is anxiety, stress, depression, or hyperactivity. In Germany, it is the main ingredient of a popular medicine, *Melissengeist,* which is prescribed for those symptoms. Taken internally for restlessness, insomnia, anxiety, headaches, depression, and heart palpitations, lemon balm is available as a dried herb, tincture, tea, capsules and oil. Teas are often combined with chamomile, valerian or passionflower for calming sleep aids. Lemon balm has no reported side effects, however, it should not be used by people with thyroid-related conditions [22].

To relieve symptoms of depression:

St. John's wort, *Hypericum perforatum:*

St. John's wort is believed to function more like the SSRIs by inhibiting the reuptake of serotonin. In laboratory studies, hyperforin, an ingredient in St. John's wort inhibits the reuptake of serotonin, dopamine, and norepinephrine[23]. According to the National Institute of Mental Health, St. John's wort may modulate the activity of interleukin-6 (Il-6), a protein involved in the communication between cells in the body's immune system. Il-6 may lead to increases in adrenal regulatory hormones a suspected cause of depression. St John's wort may reduce levels of Il-6, thus helping to ease depression [24].

Compared with the antidepressant groups, St. John's wort had lower dropout rates and numbers of patients reporting adverse effects. Eighty-one percent of the participants taking St. John's wort improved significantly, while only 26 percent of the placebo group improved. Comparative analysis of adverse effects concluded that St. John's wort seems to be at least as safe and possibly safer than conventional antidepressant drugs and is highly effective for treating mild to moderate depression, just like most antidepressants [25].

Table 7-2
Summary of Naturopathic Treatment for Bipolar Disorder [15, 16, 22] :

Common Name/ (scientific name):	Acting mechanism:	Possible side effects/ Interactions:
American Ginseng *(Panax quinquefolis)*	Active compounds of ginsenosides increases blood flow in the brain.	Toxicity side effects may include diarrhea, diminished libido, earaches, headaches, high blood pressure, insomnia, rashes, nosebleeds, vomiting. No drug interactions.
Kava kava *(Piper methysticum)*	Active compounds of kavalactones modify neurotransmitters, increases mental alertness and elevates mood.	Toxicity can cause skin, nail and hair discoloration, scaly skin, swollen eyes and face, muscle weakness, motor and vision problems. Negative interactions with alcohol, anti-anxiety and sleep medications (benzodiazepines).
Lavender *(Lavandula officinalis)*	Aromatic properties relieves stress, anxiety, insomnia, headache, nausea.	None.

Skullcap/virginian *(Scutellaria lateniflora)*	Nervous system sedative.	Toxicity could cause upset stomach, diarrhea, tics, convulsions, drowsiness. No drug interactions.
Valerian *(Valeriana officinalis)*	Central nervous system relaxant.	Toxicity may cause headache, restlessness, nausea, drowsiness, or blurred vision. Complimentary effects with prescription anti-anxiety medications.
Chamomile *(Matricaria chamomilla)*	Active ingredients of apigenin and azulene are responsible for calming the central nervous system.	Individuals with ragweed allergies may also have allergic reactions (hay fever, runny nose, congestion).
Lemon balm *(Melissa officinalis)*	Sedating action targets brain activity, frequently prescribed for insomnia, anxiety, depression, or hyperactivity.	Interactions with Thyroid medications.
Passionflower *(Passiflora incarnata)*	Alkaloids and flavonoids have sedating effects on the central nervous system.	Toxicity effects of upset stomach, nausea, vomiting, diarrhea, and sleepiness, pregnant woman should avoid. No drug interactions.
St. John's wort *(Hypericum perforatum)*	Believed to act as an anti-depressant by inhibiting the reuptake of serotonin, dopamine and norepin-phrine.	Should not be used in combination with other anti-depressants, beta-blockers, NNRTIs, seizure, heart cancer, or transplant medications.

Holistic Mental Health for Bipolar Disorder Specific Recommendations:

The mood swings of Bipolar Disorder can be very serious, and treatment whether it be traditional or alternative should be under the care of a physician. A naturopathetic physician may suggest the following in addition to the above suggestions:

- Eat an organic diet with foods such as whole grains, vegetables, fruits and fish. Drink only spring water.

- Eliminate processed foods from the diet (any with foods with chemical additives). Restrict sugar, and caffeine in the diet.

- Take a multi-vitamin/mineral daily with additional vitamin C (2-3,000 mg, per day) B-Complex (100 mg 2 times per day), vitamin E (400-800 IU's per day), calcium (1,200-1,500 mg, per day), magnesium (600-800 mg, per day) selenium (75-100 mcg, per day), zinc (30-40 mg, per day).

- Additional essential fatty acids should be taken by eating cold water fish (salmon, tuna) or taking an Alpha-linclenic acid supplement.

- Use aromatherapy at home by using scented oils, bath oils or soaps such as Lavender, Melissa or Rose. Try yoga or spend time each day in meditation.

- Get a therapeutic massage with essential oils such as Clary sage, Lavender, Melissa, Rose, or Ylang-Ylang.

Treatment for medical conditions should always be conducted by your healthcare professional. According to the FDA only physicians are allowed to prescribe medications, and the suggestions in this book are for dietary changes and/or supplements only.

Schizophrenia

Most people think of delusions such as hearing voices or seeing imaginary people or animals when they hear of schizophrenia. However, delusions may or may not be a symptom of the disorder. It is believed about 1 percent of the population may suffer from Schizophrenia. Typically, symptoms begin in late adolescents or early adulthood. Men and woman share the frequency of the disorder, however, woman usually have a 5 year later onset of the disorder.

Symptoms of Schizophrenia were first categorized in 1856 by Morel, who was treating an adolescent boy. At that time he termed the disorder *precocious dementia*. It wasn't until the early 1900's did the term Schizophrenia replace Morel's name. Bleuler developed the name Schizophrenia after observing that the symptoms do not usually lead to mental deterioration as in other forms of dementia [26].

Recent studies on the likelihood of schizophrenia occurring estimates that the disorder affects 7 to 8 individuals out of 1,000. The study from the University of Queensland, in Australia, reviewed 188 studies on schizophrenia from 46 countries. Among their findings:

- Schizophrenia is more common in developed countries than in developing nations.

- Similar rates of schizophrenia were seen among men and women, as well as urban and rural residents.

- Schizophrenia rates were nearly twice as high for immigrants as for native-born people [27].

The DSM-IV classifies Schizophrenia as a psychotic disorder with a number of variations based on the symptoms. A common characteristic of Schizophrenia, Schizophreniform Disorder, Schizoaffective Disorder, and Brief Psychotic Disorder, are psychotic delusions, any prominent hallucinations, disorganized speech, and disorganized or catatonic behavior.

Definitions of the disorders in this category [28]:

Schizophrenia: Lasts for at least 6 months and includes at least one month of active symptoms; two or more of the following: delusions, hallucinations, disorganized speech, grossly disorganized or catatonic behavior, negative symptoms.

Schizophreniform Disorder: similar symptoms to that of Schizophrenia but with shorter duration (1 to 6 months), and the absence that there be a decline in functioning.

Schizoaffective Disorder: is a disorder in which a mood episode and the active-phase symptoms of Schizophrenia occur together and were preceded or are followed by at least 2 weeks of delusions or hallucinations without prominent mood symptoms.

Delusional Disorder: characterized by at least one month of no bizarre delusions without other active-phrase symptoms of Schizophrenia.

Brief Psychotic Disorder: a disorder that lasts for more than one day, and remits by one month.

Shared Psychotic Disorder: characterized by the presence of a delusion in an individual who is influenced by someone else who has a longer-standing delusion with similar content.

Causes of Schizophrenia:

Brain Abnormalities

Over the past hundred years several theories have emerged as to the cause of Schizophrenia. Magnetic resonance imaging (MRI) and computed tomography (CT) brain scans have supported some theories of brain abnormalities in Schizophrenic patients. Research has shown that 50 percent of patients with Schizophrenia have enlarged ventricles. Temporal lobe differences has also been noted. Normally the left temporal lobe of the brain is larger than the right, however, in schizophrenia the right has been noted to be larger. Decreased size due to neuron loss, quite possibly from viral infections has also been seen in the hippocampus in Schizophrenia patients. The hippocampus is involved in memory and learning, which is usually diminished in schizophrenia.

Scientists have also observed diminished size of brain cortices for the past hundred years in individuals with Schizophrenia. On the average a 5 percent reduction in brain weight and a 7 percent decrease in cortical thickness has been observed. Negative symptoms such as cognitive slowing, apathy, withdrawal, inappropriate or flatten affect can be connected to this decrease in prefrontal cortex size. Schizophrenia patients may also have reduced blood flow to the brain (hypometabolic state) that is thought to contribute to diminished higher cognitive tasks such as abstract thought, goal setting, spontaneity and short-term memory [29].

The effect certain psychotic medications has on Schizophrenia patients leads to neurochemical theories of the cause of the disorder. By giving patients dopamine inhibiting drugs such as chlorpromazine is was observed that symptoms such as hallucinations an delusions diminished. Therefore, many researchers believe that symptoms are caused by an increased level of dopamine in the brain. Research indicates that a decrease in Glutamate, an excitatory neurotransmitter, exists in individuals with Schizophrenia. Decreased Glutamate could be responsible for flatten cognitive processes. GABA is an inhibitory neurotransmitter, and there is evidence that suggests that individuals with Schizophrenia have unusually low levels of this amino acid. Inadequate inhibition in the frontal cortex related to decreased levels of GABA may account for the loss of filtering and selective attention (inability to ignore unimportant stimulation such as background noise), that is often a symptom of Schizophrenia.

Genetics

In addition to the genetic implications from the Swedish study (Genetic causes of bipolar disorder), researchers in New York believe they have found a DNA evidence that may indicate a higher risk for schizophrenia. They found a higher incidence of a two genes: CSF2RA and IL3RA on individuals with schizophrenia [30].

Researchers from Cambridge, England's Babraham Institute found that genes that are responsible for producing the protective coating around nerves in the brains of the people with disorders like schizophrenia and bipolar disorder were less active than people without these disorders. Professor Kenneth Davis, MD says that this research has prompted a sea of change over the cause of schizophrenia. He stated that everyone had thought schizophrenia was related to nerve cells and signal transmission in the brain, not myelin (nerve cell coverings). Researchers now know that these myelin genes are less active, and we need to find out why [31].

Health Causes

Prenatal health may have a link to the incidence of schizophrenia. A study from Columbia University found that the risk of developing schizophrenia was three times higher among adult children exposed to influenza during the first half of pregnancy, compared to those who had not been exposed. If the mothers were exposed during the first trimester, the incidence of developing schizophrenia was seven times higher. However, if mothers were exposed to the flu in the second half of their pregnancy there was no increased risk associated [32].

Stress may be a factor that may worsen disorders like bipolar disorder and schizophrenia. Studies from Yale University with animals found that stress increases a protein kinase C or PKC in the brain. They found that excessive PKC activation can disrupt the regulation of thought in the prefrontal cortex of the brain. This can lead to though disorders, impaired judgment, distractibility and impulsivity [33].

Summer births have been linked to a higher incidence of *deficit* schizophrenia. Deficit schizophrenia is a sub-type of schizophrenia that has symptoms of social withdrawal, depression, and apathy. A study in the *Archives of General Psychiatry* (2004) of 1,594 patients with schizophrenia living in Ireland, England, Scotland, Spain and the U.S., found that more patients were born in June and July that had schizophrenia then any other month of the year. Researchers believe that factors contributing to this could be sunlight exposure, vitamin D and infectious agents [34].

Gluten intolerance has also been linked to schizophrenia. Researchers from John's Hopkins University found that people with a genetic digestive disorder known as celiac disease were three times more likely than the general population to develop schizophrenia. Celiac disease is a condition in which foods that contain gluten damage the small intestine. This damage makes it hard for the body to absorb nutrients, especially fat, calcium, iron, and folate from food. Researchers state that the next step would to determine if a gluten-free diet makes a difference in the symptoms of schizophrenic people with celiac disease [35].

Carl Pfeiffer, M.D., director of the Brain Bio in Skillman, NJ who has been involved in psychiatric research for over 50 years believes that there are a number of biological and environmental factors that could contribute to schizophrenic symptoms. He believes Schizophrenia could be caused by: vitamin deficiencies, drug intoxications, sleep deprivation, heavy metal toxicity, hypoglycemia, cerebral allergies, food sensitivities, pyroluria, chronic candida infection, Huntington's chorea, and Wilson's disease [36].

Allopathic Treatment for Schizophrenia:

Antipsychotic medications are usually prescribed for Schizophrenia. Since the first, chlorpromazine was introduced in public hospitals (1954) there has been a dramatic decrease of psychiatric patients committed to state hospitals. In 1955 more than 558,000 were in state hospitals, by 1997 that number has dropped by 85 percent to approximately 70,000. Many patients are living and functioning in the community today due to the treatment they receive from medications. However, most medications carry with them significant side-effects.

Categories of medications that are used for Schizophrenia include:

Traditional agents; (High-potency drugs) Fluphenazine (*Prolixin*), Haloperidol (*Haldol*), Thiothixene (*Navane*), Trifluoperazine (*Stelazine*), (Moderate-potency drugs) Loxapine (*Loxitane*), Molindone (*Moban*), Perphenazine (*Taractan*), (Low-potency drugs) Chlorpromazine (*Thorazine*).

Atypical Agents; Clozapine (*Clozaril*), Olanzapine (*Zyprexa*), Quatrain (*Seroquel*), Risperidone (*Risperdal*). See *Table 7-3* for these medications and possible side-effects.

Table 7-3
Summary of Allopathic Treatment for Schizophrenia [25]:

Drug: (brand name)	*Acting mechanism:*	*Possible side effects:*
Antipsychotics: **Areipiprazole** (*Abilify*), **Clozapine** (*Clorazil*), **Olanzapine** (*Symbyax, Zyprexa*), **Quatrain** (*Seroquel*), **Risperidone** (*Risperdal, Risperdal Consta,*), **Ziprasidone** (*Geodon*)	It appears to alleviate symptoms of mania by blocking certain nerve impulses between nerve cells.	Abdominal pain, abnormal gait, agitation, anxiety, back pain, behavior problems, blood in urine, blurred vision, chest pain, constipation, dehydration, dizziness, drowsiness, dry mouth, skin or eyes, extreme low or high blood pressure, fever, headache, insomnia, joint pain, involuntary movements, muscle rigidity, nausea, nervousness, tremors, weight gain, sexual dysfunction, stroke, heart attack.

Phenothiazines: **Fluphenazine** (*Prolixin*), **Perphenazine** (*Taractan*), **Chlorpromazine** (*Thorazine*), **Trifluoperazine** (*Stelazine*)	Suppresses brain centers responsible for abnormal emotions and behaviors, also suppresses brain's vomiting reflect center.	Dry mouth, blurred vision, constipation, difficulty urinating, sedation, dizziness, low blood pressure, involuntary movements, tremor, muscle rigidity, restlessness, muscle spasms, jaundice, high fever, rapid pulse, confusion, irritability, seizures.
Haloperidol: (*Haldol, Halperon Novo-Peridol, Peridol, PMS- Haloperidol*)	Blocks dopamine, corrects an imbalance in nerve impulses in the brain.	Involuntary movements, tremor, muscle rigidity, restlessness, muscle spasms of the face, eyes tongue, jaw, neck, body or limbs, high fever, rapid pulse, confusion, irritability, seizures.
Thiothixene: (*Navane, Thiothixene HCI, Intensol*)	Corrects imbalance of nerve impulses.	Sedation, dizziness, low blood pressure, involuntary movements, tremor, muscle rigidity, restlessness, muscle spasms, jaundice, high fever, rapid pulse, confusion, irritability, seizures.
Loxapine: (*Loxitane, Loxapac, Loxitane- C*)	Blocks the effect of dopamine in the brain.	Dry mouth, decreased salivation, swallowing difficulty, lack of expression, muscle rigidity, dizziness, tremor, constipation, urination difficulty, blurred vision, confusion, loss of sex drive, headache, insomnia, menstrual irregularities, weight gain, light sensitivity, nausea, shortness of breath, skin rash, irregular heartbeat, profuse sweating, fever, convulsions.
Molindone: (*Moban, Moban Concentrate*)	Corrects imbalance of nerve impulses in the brain.	Involuntary movements, sedation, low blood pressure, dizziness, tremor, muscle rigidity, restlessness, muscle spasms of the face, eyes tongue, jaw, neck, body or limbs, high fever, rapid pulse, confusion, irritability, seizures.

Naturopathic Therapy for Schizophrenia:

Dr. Carl Pfeiffer and the Brain Bio Center in New Jersey had studied mental disorders, and particularly Schizophrenia for over 50 years. He and his Center have developed treatments for mental disorders based on nutritional deficiencies individuals may have. After treating thousands of patients diagnosed with Schizophrenia he determined there are five main "biotypes" based on their blood work:

Histapenia: Low blood histamine with excess copper; 50 percent of Schizophrenics.

Histadelia: High blood histamine with low copper; 20 percent of Schizophrenics.

Pyroluria: A familial double deficiency of zinc and vitamin B_6; 30 percent of Schizophrenics.

Cerebral Allergy: Includes wheat-gluten allergy; 10 percent of Schizophrenics.

Nutritional Hypoglycemia: 20 percent of Schizophrenics.

The above percentages do not add up to 100 percent due to the fact that many individuals observed had multiple disorders contributing to their Schizophrenic symptoms [37].

Histamine is chemical that can cross the blood-brain barrier and is found in the brain in low quantities. It is believed to react on neurons in the hypothalamus region in the brain and extend to many Central Nervous System (CNS) areas. The receptors for histamine initiate secondary messenger transmission. Histamine is also believed to be involved in body functions such as the regulation of biorhythms, thermoregulation, and in neuroendrocrine functions. Histamine may be excitatory or inhibitory depending on the action of the receptors involved [38].

Dr. Pfeiffer describes the **histapenic** patient as being low in histamine and having excess copper in the tissues. This combination can cause behavioral abnormalities consistent with Schizophrenia symptoms such as hallucinations, paranoia, and anxiety. Increased copper may be caused from household copper water pipes and copper cookware. Other environmental toxins found in excess in Schizophrenia patients includes iron, mercury and lead, all considered toxic heavy metals. Essential trace elements such as manganese and zinc are lower than normal in Schizophrenia patients. Histapenic individuals may have:

- Canker sores
- Ringing in the ears
- Heavy growth of body hair
- Excess fat in the lower extremities
- Difficult orgasm in sex
- Ideas of grandeur
- Undue suspicion of people
- The feeling that someone controls your mind
- Seeing or hearing things abnormally
- The ability to endure pain well
- No headaches or allergies

Dr. Pfeiffer recommended the following for histapenic patients:

- Niacin; 100 mg in morning and in the evening
- niacin amide; 250-500 mg in the morning and evening
- Folic acid; 1,000 mcg in the morning
- B_{12} injection, weekly or in a daily supplementation
- L-tryptophan; 1,000 mg in the evening
- Zinc and manganese daily
- High protein diet [39].

Too much histamine can cause allergic reactions. depression, hyperactivity or compulsive behaviors. High levels of histamine, histaldelic, in the body is usually an inherited trait. Characteristics of an individual with **histaldelic** could include:

Dr. Pfeiffer recommended the following for histaldelic patients:

- A low protein diet, and a high complex carbohydrate diet
- Calcium (as gluconate); 500 mg, in morning and evening
- Methionine; 500 mg morning and evening [40].

Pyrroles are a chemical compound that were first connected with psychosis in 1958, when Canadian researchers first noted a substance in the urine of patients undergoing experimental LSD model psychosis. It was also found in psychiatric patients that have never taken LSD. This compound was also found to deplete the body of B_6 and zinc. Dr. Pfeiffer found that 30 percent of Schizophrenic patients have pryroluria. Symptoms of a pyroluric individual includes:

- Difficulty with perception and:
- Intolerance to some protein foods and alcohol
- Definite breath and body order
- Morning nausea and constipation, frequent upper abdominal pain
- Difficulty in remembering dreams
- Crowded upper front teeth
- White spots on your finger nails
- Pale skin that does not tolerate sunlight well
- Frequent head colds and infections
- Stretch marks in the skin
- Irregular menstrual cycle or impotency
- Any of the above when stressed
- You belong to an all girl family, with look-alike sisters.

Dr. Pfeiffer suggested the following for his pyroluric patients:

Vitamin B_6 ; in the morning, enough for nightly dream recall (do not exceed 2,000 mg)
Zinc; 30 mg, morning and evening
Manganese; 10 mg in the morning and evening [41].

Cerebral allergies are similar to traditional allergies such as hay fever that "run" in a family. Dr. Pfeiffer describe cerebral allergies as having symptoms of irritability, hyperactivity, impaired concentration and Schizophrenic symptoms in severe cases. It is most often caused by intolerance to certain foods such as: food dyes and additives, milk, wheat, eggs, beef, corn, cane sugar, and chocolate. The individual often does not know they are intolerant or allergic to certain foods, and may even crave them. Cerebral allergies may express the following symptoms:

- Difficulty with perception and:
- A history of infantile colic or eczema
- A history of celiac disease, rashes, asthma or hay fever
- Frequent colds and seasonal allergies
- Excessive daily mood swings
- Intolerance to foods such as wheat or milk
- Relief of symptoms when fasting

For individuals with cerebral allergies the following is recommended:

- Methionine; 500 mg morning and evening
- Calcium; 500 mg morning and evening
- Zinc; 15 mg morning and evening
- Manganese; 10 mg morning and evening
- B_6 ; adequate for dream recall (do not exceed 2,000 mg)
- Vitamin C; 1,000 to 2,000 mg morning and evening
- An organic diet; eliminate any foods with additives such as food dyes and preservatives. Eliminate aspirin and foods with salicylates (see ADHD chapter) [42].

Psychosis and Schizophrenia can occur when the blood-sugar balance in the brain is out of balance. **Nutritional Hypoglycemia** (low blood sugar) and diabetes (high blood sugar) can result in the signs and symptoms of mental imbalance. Glucose imbalance or intolerance may have symptoms such as:

- Difficulty with perception and:
- Weakness, fatigue, faintness, and dizziness

- Nervousness, irritability, trembling, and anxiety
- Depression, forgetfulness, confusion, and difficulty concentrating
- Palpitations or blackouts

Dr. Pfeiffer recommended the following:

- Avoidance of junk foods, sugar, alcohol and white bread
- Regular exercise
- Manganese; 10 mg in morning and evening
- Zinc; 15 mg in morning and evening
- B_3 and chromium; in morning and evening
- A multi-vitamin without copper [43].

In addition to Dr. Pfeiffer's above nutritional therapies for Schizophrenia a number of calming herbs could be beneficial. Research supports the use of several herbs that have similar properties and calming effects as prescription medications, without the side effects. **American ginseng** contains ginsenosides that is believed to reduce stress and anxiety by reducing blood flow to the brain. Side effects have only been observed when excessive amounts have used.

Kava is another herb that has been used for centuries to treat anxiety and stress. Kavalactones, the active ingredient in Kava is believed to work by modifying action of neurotransmitters, creating a calming effect. Side effects of Kava are reported with high doses.

Valerian, a herb that has been used for over 1,000 years as a calming sleep aid has been proven to be effective in treating anxiety, stress-related headaches, tension and insomnia. Unlike prescription sedatives it does not interfere with sleep cycles. Side effects have been observed with over consumption or when used in combination with prescription tranquilizers.

Other less "clinically" studied herbs that have been reported to have calming effects on the nervous system include **Lavender**, an aromatic herb that is used internally, externally and in aromatherapy, **Skullcap/Virginian**, used as a sedative and digestive aid, **Chamomile**, used as a central nervous system sedative, **Lemon Balm,** also sedating and will relieve indigestion, and **Passionflower**, used for chronic stress relief, anxiety and insomnia [44].

Holistic Mental Health for Schizophrenia Specific Recommendations:

Consultation with a naturopathetic physician is recommended that can conduct blood, urine and allergy tests to determine the type of Schizophrenia. A naturopathetic physician may suggest the following in addition to the above suggestions:

- Eliminate toxins from the environment and food supply by eating an organic diet with foods such as whole grains, vegetables, fruits and fish. Drink only spring water.

- Eliminate processed foods from the diet (any with foods with chemical additives). Eliminate any foods with additives such as food dyes and preservatives. Eliminate aspirin and foods with calculates. Eliminate sugar, alcohol, and caffeine in the diet.

- Follow specific vitamin and mineral supplementations above based on type of Schizophrenia.

- Use calming herbs such as American Ginseng, Kava kava, Valerian, Skullcap, Lavender, or Chamomile.

- Consultation with a spiritual healer to determine if supernatural influences may be a factor (see chapter VII).

Treatment for medical conditions should always be conducted by your healthcare professional. According to the FDA only physicians are allowed to prescribe medications, and the suggestions in this book are for dietary changes and/or supplements only.

CHAPTER VIII:
SPIRITUAL HEALING

I have sticker on a file cabinet in my office that I got from a conference somewhere 5 or 6 years ago that says *"Change your mind about mental illness."* Little did I know how true that would become. I, like most psychologists would not give a second thought to referring a patient for further help such as looking into medication, or even hospitalization, if someone came into my office telling me they were hearing voices or seeing spirits.

However, when you have been around people that can see energy in forms that we would call spirits, that can heal with a wave of their hands, or that can tell you what you did in a past life, your perspective on what might be real or imagined changes. Granted having a background in hypnotherapy I have regressed patients into past lives and I do believe in reincarnation. And, I have even had some personal experiences that I consider paranormal. But what I have experienced in the last few years go far beyond what you can learn from textbooks.

Paranormal Coincidences?

When I was a child we lived about 2 hours away from my grandmother's house in Rhode Island. One morning, my mother awoke saying she had a dream that there was a fire in her mother's house. Of course she called to check, and surprisingly there had been a fire the night before. No one was hurt but my grandmother's house was destroyed.

Years later my mother was suffering from advanced Alzheimer's she was bedridden and totally unresponsive. She was being cared for by my stepfather who in fact had to do everything for her, just as one would have to care for a newborn baby. I had visited a week before and noticed no change in her situation. She had been in the same state of health for the past two years, and we expected her to be that way for many more years. One Saturday morning I awoke from a very vivid dream. My family and I were taking a walk on a dirt road through the woods. My stepfather was leading with my brother and sisters behind him, I was about 10 yards further back and my mother was walking some 20 yards further behind me. It was getting dark and I turned to my mother and said "come on mom you'll get lost." She looked at me and said "You go on without me, I'll be O.K."

That morning I woke up to my stepfather calling to tell me my mother had died that night. It wasn't a case that anyone had expected her to die. Or, that I had even checked in the night before to see how she was doing. I felt her death was virtually "out of the blue." And, I know in my heart, and soul, she had talked to me that night before as she transitioned to the spirit world.

This experience confirmed to me that there is psychic energy that transcends us. I realize that most scientists would dismiss an event such as my mother talking to me in a dream before she died as just a coincidence. However, I have since been with people who talk to "spirits" in the waking state.

Spiritual Awakening

Through my wife's spiritual awakening in the last few years (enough information for another book) we have met people that could see and use energy that others can't. People that can talk to spirits, tell you of your past and of your future. And heal others using energy fields.

I have come to understand that those people have gifts. And, in talking with many of them they realized at a young age that they were different from other people. They could see energy or spirits, or hear things others couldn't since childhood. Parents that do not have such gifts would often try to dismiss their child's claims of seeing or hearing things to their imagination. And, if their child persisted they might bring them to a professional. And a psychiatrist would surely have an array of drugs that can suppress those sights or voices (and probably diagnose them as schizophrenic).

Grace was one of my first, firsthand encounters with such a gifted individual. I came into contact with her when my wife and I where running out of medical explanations for her continued gastrointestinal difficulties. My wife Mary had been in the hospital with severe stomach cramps and bloating; and had had every test doctors could think of. All tests came back perfectly normal. No colon abnormalities, no ulcers, all internal organs perfectly normal, blood pressure, antibodies and all other metabolic rates, all perfectly normal. Yet her cramps and bloating persisted. Her skin was becoming dry and flaky and her lips felt like they were on fire.

A few months before Mary had been getting sick she had gone into a little holistic herb and gift shop called *Herbs and Angels*. There she notice an array of healing herbs, and spiritual gifts, jewelry and books. We thought perhaps something there might help. Walking into the shop we met a woman whose name was Grace, that we later learned was, in every sense of the word. Grace took one look at Mary and told her, "You have an entity in you!" Mary's reaction was one of relief. She told Grace "I thought I had something in me." Grace then ushered Mary into a back room where she could work on her.

When they emerged, close to an hour later, Mary looked significantly better. However, Grace felt that there was several layers of energy or entities attacking Mary and suggested more sessions with her. I was initially apprehensive. Did Grace really get rid of "evil spirits" causing the discomfort in my wife? Could she really see spirits or layers of energy? Or, was Mary feeling better simply through the power of suggestion from Grace (as in hypnosis)? Or, was Grace setting us up to "scam" more money out of us?

But then again, Mary was feeling much better after just one session with Grace, so we arranged to have another session with her next week. In the meantime, Grace had called her mentor, Alan because she later told us that she had never come across someone like Mary. She told us that most of her patients are cleared after one session. Grace had never seen anyone with so much energy built up in them as what she saw in Mary. The next week both Alan and Grace worked on releasing these entities from Mary. And, Mary got better and better each week.

One time when Grace had come to our house to work on Mary, somewhat out of the blue, Grace looked in my direction and said "I feel a lot of love around you. There is a short stocky woman with dark hair who is by your side. She is a very strong woman. I believe she was your grandmother." Now, I had only known Grace for a few weeks. I had never discussed my family with her. I did not have any family pictures out that she could have seen. And I, nor did Mary, ever tell Grace that my grandmother had died 5 years ago. Yet, she described her perfectly. My apprehension about her abilities and possible questionable intensions was diminishing.

In talking further to Grace and Alan about their work, we came to find out that although Grace was able to see spirits and energy fields since she was a child she was now an apprentice of Alan's who also had these abilities. Alan was in the business of healing people by releasing these negative attachments. He told us that occasionally when someone dies they do not crossover immediately to the "light." That they get confused or trapped in the earthly dimersion. And, they can attach themselves to someone causing a number of problems for their hosts!

These lost entities can cause the person they are attached to, to be anxious, depressed and even violently sick. Alan and Grace explained that they are attracted to someone's energy field . They usually don't even know that they are deceased. When Alan and Grace are working with someone that has one or more of these entities attached to them they are able to cross them over to the light so they can transition into the spirit realm. In working with Mary they were continually crossing over entities. Alan explained that she had many layers of these entities attached to her for some time. Due to Mary's high Vibrational energy these entities thought she was the light.

Over the next few years several people we came into contact with that could see or feel energy told Mary that she has incredible vibrational energy also. The result of Alan and Grace's healings was that Mary was feeling better every week.

These events were just the beginning of Mary's spiritual awakening. Mary began seeing energy fields herself. They were not the steady images that Grace saw, but quick glimpse of someone's face changing into someone else's. Initially this was very unnerving to Mary. She would scream when she saw these images (unnerving for me also when she would scream every time she saw me!). However, after working with Grace and Alan after she began calming down and was able to focus on the images. We have come to believe that these images Mary sees in people's faces are often the faces of their past lives.

Worlds we Never Dreamed of

Mary was also led to others that have had similar experiences (although not as physically dramatic) to hers. When conducting a search on the internet, she was led to Dr. Michael Sharp, author of a number of books on spiritual awakening (see suggested readings). Through him we began learning more about energy fields around our bodies called chakras, about universal energies, and about ancient civilizations that were connected to these energies and were able to do amazing things. We were lead to Gregg Braden author of *The Divine Matrix*, and *Walking Between Worlds,* who describes coming through the darkness, about ancient messages, 2012, and connecting to universal energies.

She was led to people that use these chakras and energy fields to heal. Peggy Phoenix Dubro, describes how to use bands of energy around the body to heal in her book *Elegant Empowerment.* As does Caroline Myss, Ph.D. in

Anatomy of the Spirit, Richard Gerber, M.D. in *Vibrational Medicine, New Choices for Healing Ourselves,* Julie Motz in *Hands of Life,* and Barbara Ann Brennan in *Hands of Light, A Guide to Healing Through the Human Energy Field.* And, Dr. Eric Pearl, author of *The Reconnection* who uses a universal frequency that has resulted in miraculous healings (www.TheReconnection. com)

We have met other people that connect to the spirit realm and have written about it. People like Lee Carroll who in his *Kryon* series of books, channels a master spirit. Esther and Jerry Hicks channel a master spirit named Abraham. Doreen Virtue, Ph.D. writes about connecting with guardian angels, and Sonia Choquette tells you how to connect with your guides, to name a few.

We have come into contact with people that discuss universal energy shifts that are in process and will continue through the year 2012. Authors such as Drunvalo Melchizedek in his books *Serpent of Light, Beyond 2012,* and *The Ancient Secret of the Flower of Life,* and Barbara Hand Clow in her book *The Mayan Code,* both describe this global energy transformation that we are in the process of going through now and beyond the year 2012.

The Age of New Age

The above authors are just a few of the *New Age* authors and speakers of the past ten years that have come into national prominence. This gradual national and world-wide awakening has been aided by people like Louise Hay author of the book and movie *You Can Heal Your Life.* And by her publishing house, Hay House that supports new age authors and sponsors speaking events worldwide. People like Oprah Winfrey that have had many of these authors on her show. By a number of TV shows centered around clairvoyant individuals solving crimes and helping people. Shows like *Ghost Hunters, Supernatural, The Ghost Whisper, Medium, The Mentalist, The Dead Zone,* and movies like the *Sixth Sense* are getting the public to gradually accept that some people have special gifts, and are able to see and talk to spirits. And, the internet is linking the world together with authors and people that can heal with energy or talk to your guides and guardian angels.

The *New Age* movement can also be called the *"Ancient New."* In the late 1960's I was led to a series of books by Carlos Castaneda that described his experiences and subsequent apprenticeship with an Yaqui Indian shaman named Don Juan Matus. What turned into a series of 12 books over nearly 30 years described extraordinary abilities of the Indian Shaman. From reading the series is was evident that Don Juan had the ability to not only see energy fields but was able to manipulate them. He was able to change his physical appearance, to connect with universal energies, see beings from other dimensions, and foretell future events.

Twenty years before Carlos Castaneda's books Paramhansa Yogananda in *The Autobiography of a Yogi* (1946) describes similar feats of yogi masters from India. Paramhansa through his life-long pursuit of becoming a yogi master himself, describes meetings with other masters that could also change their appearance, levitate, transcend space and time and communicate with the spirit world.

In the 1920's Ernest Holmes, an international authority on religious psychology, founder of the Religious Science movement, and author of a number of books including *The Science of Mind* (1926) discuses concepts that are continually expounded on by new age authors and motivational speakers. Concepts like the power of meditation, connecting with spirit, the infinite, the God Source of the universe. He describes how thoughts have substance and create intent, that thoughts can do anything one desires. How thoughts can heal the body connect one to the source, change one's life. Sound familiar? Perhaps like a new age or motivational speaker?

One of the greatest new agers, or ancient new, shaman, yogi master that ever lived was Jesus. Over two thousand years ago he was doing yogi master and shaman-like feats. By connecting to the *God-Source* he was able to turn water into wine, walk on water, and raise the dead. And, did he not state that by believing as he does you can do what he does? How's that for connecting with spirit, positive intent, and changing one's life by changing your thoughts?

Religion and Reincarnation

A theme every religion has, since the beginning of recorded time is belief in an afterlife. That we have a soul and it goes somewhere (like heaven) after we die. I have always felt that since we do have a soul, and it is eternal, and that if we go somewhere after we die, then we must have come from somewhere before we were born. Religions like Buddhism believes in, and promotes reincarnation. That by leading a good life your next life will be better. And, that by learning and growing in each subsequent life you grow your soul until you reach enlightenment like Buddha did.

Early Christian beliefs promoted the idea of reincarnation. References to reincarnation have been found in the Old and New Testaments. However, during the Second Council of Constantinople, in the year 553 a.d., the concept of reincarnation was declared to be a heresy. The church at that time felt that the concept of multiple lives would give individuals too much time for salvation and would undermine the growing power of the church.

Unfortunately, the Catholic Church didn't see at that time that fundamental questions of why we are here, can be answered by the Buddhist philosophy and through reincarnation. Buddhists believe we are here to learn and grow our soul. The more pain, hardships and even suffering one goes through in life, the more their soul grows. This is a great philosophy that more people believe in worldwide than don't. But, getting back to science how do you prove reincarnation?

Proving Reincarnation

As previously mentioned in my private practice I use hypnotherapy. I have regressed individuals into past lives, and I have been regressed myself into past lives. So I do believe in reincarnation. And, the Buddhist philosophy makes perfect sense to me. We are here to learn and grow our souls. Our life, the family we are born into, the people we meet and travel with, and the events in our life, are all designed to grow our souls.

But the most pressing question in the field of past life regression is how do you prove it? Are the visions someone is having when they are "under" real or imagined? If after the regression, the patient tells of living in the American old west, and that her name was Samuel Johnson. And she was killed in an Indian raid while traveling through the Arizona territory in 1820. Or, that she was a princess in England that died when having a child in the 1400's. How do you prove these claims? And even if there were records how do you know that she didn't read about these people at some point in her life? Even when she was a child in elementary school and these stories were buried deep within her subconscious, only to emerge when hypnotized. This has been the controversy in past life regression, are the events recalled real or imagined? And how do you prove them?

As far as I am concerned a number of researchers have *proved* reincarnation. Ian Stevenson, M.D., Professor of Psychiatry at the University of Virginia went about researching claims of reincarnation primarily with children. He documented over two thousand instances where children recalled reincarnation-type memories. They would recall places were they lived, being able to describe towns and even layouts of houses, as well as names of places and people they lived with. They were able to speak languages not exposed to in their present life. Dr. Stevenson researched these claims and verified that they were true. The only explanation was that these children had in fact lived in these places before they were born into their present life.

Two other individuals have also collected an overwhelming body of evidence proving reincarnation exists through the use of hypnotherapy. Michael Newton, Ph.D. and Brain Weiss, M.D. have documented thousands of cases of individuals reporting past life experiences. Michael Newton author of *Journey of Souls, Life Between Lives* and *Destiny of Souls* not only regressed people into past lives, but he had them talk about the time between lives. Where they were before they were born. Their "life' in the spirit realm.

Dr. Weiss was chief resident in psychiatry at Yale University School of Medicine and later Chairman of the Department of Psychiatry at Mount Sinai Medical Center in Miami, Fl, and is author of best selling books such as *Many Lives, Many Masters,* and *Messages from the Masters.* And, like Dr. Newton, Dr. Weiss was amazed when patients started telling him of previous lives and experiences of being in the spirit world.

What constitutes scientific fact? In clinical trails a significant percentage has to be achieved in order for results to be verified. In a scientific study when the same results are achieved over and over again a scientific theory or principle is formulated. The key being that the same results can be duplicated. Much like the when you drop something. You can be pretty certain that because of the principle of gravity that it will fall to the earth. If you regress 1 or 2 or 6 people to the time between their lives and they tell you similar stories, well that might be coincidence. Popular beliefs about what the spirit world might be like, could explain how these 6 people came up with similar stories. However, when you regress thousands of people from all different walks of life, from all different ethnic and religious backgrounds, and they tell you the same stories of what the spirit world is like you have clinically significant evidence that this is a scientific principle (or a universal principle).

This is what Dr. Stevenson, Dr. Newton and Dr. Weiss describe. *Clinical evidence* that reincarnation exists. Many different researchers, conducting thousands of "tests or experiments", arriving at the same conclusions or results, constitutes *clinical evidence.* And, what they have found are facts like: we plan the life we come into, who we will become, the family we will be part of, who we will marry. That we travel from life to life with the same people that make-up our *soul groups.* That many of the challenges in life, be it physical, emotional, or relational, are ones we put in our life in order to grow our souls!

What does this all have to do with one's mental health? Adults should realize that when children describe living with other people in other places that they are most likely recalling a past life. When you have a *déjà vu* experience about a place or person, that you are recalling a past life experience. That when you have a challenge in life, you most likely placed it there so you can learn and grow from it. That your loved ones never really leave you. Death is only a physical body occurrence. Our souls are eternal. Making us spiritual beings having a physical experience.

Holistic Mental Health for
Spiritual Health
Specific Recommendations:

If someone that is hearing voices or seeing "ghosts" (as long as there is no danger to harm oneself or others) do not be too quick to hospitalize them or place them on mind-numbing drugs.

- When experiencing supernatural events like hearing voices or seeing energy, consult with a lightworker (someone that is reputable, and that can themselves, connect with spiritual energy).

- If experiencing physical pain that cannot be medically diagnosed seek out a spiritual healer.

- Read books like *Destiny of Souls* by Michael Newton, and *Messages from the Masters* by Brian Weiss, to gain an understanding of why we are here and why things happen in our lives.

*"With the realization of ones own potential
and self confidence in one's ability,
one can build a better world."*
~ Dalai Lama

CHAPTER IX:
Conclusions and Implications

As the debate rages on between the type of treatment to use for mental disorders it appears that individuals do have viable options. Mental disorders such as Alzheimer's disease, anxiety, stress, ADHD, depression, headaches and migraines, bipolar disorder and schizophrenia, all have several treatment options both in allopathic and naturopathic medicine.

The primary difference between the two approaches appears to be whether to treat the symptoms or the cause of the disorder. Allopathic treatment focuses more on treating the symptoms with various medications until the illness dissipates. Naturopathic treatment places more emphasis on finding the cause of the disorder, and preventing the illness from continuing.

CHAPTER SUMMARIES:

Alzheimer's Disease

Alzheimer's Disease (AD) is the most common form of dementia affecting an estimated 5 million individuals in the U.S., increasing in prevalence from 6 percent at age 65, to 41 percent in females at age 95 [1]. Alzheimer's Disease is believed to be caused by a variety of factors. High aluminum concentrations are believed to effect the neurotransmitter, acetylcholine and acts as a neurotoxin impairing chemical reactions in the brain[2]. A possible genetic defect can lead to an over production of interleukin-6 that stimulates production of beta amyloid that causes free radical damage to neurons in the brain[3]. Other environmental toxins such as lead and zinc have been shown to be in high concentration of patients with AD [4].

Allopathic treatment for AD uses estrogen replacement therapy or an array of newer drugs. Estrogen replacement therapy or hormone replacement therapy (HRT) was originally thought to slow down the effects of AD, however, the use of HRT has been reported to increase the risk of breast cancer. Other side effects may include irregular bleeding, fluid retention, breast tenderness and headaches. Serious side effects could include uterine cancer, heart problems, gallbladder disease, and increased blood clotting[5]. Newer prescription medications for AD increase the brain's supply of acetycholine, include physostigmine, tacrine, donepezil, metrifonate, revastigmine, and eptastigmine. All of which have been shown to improve memory and cognition in trials. Side effects of these medications could include nausea, dizziness, vomiting, diarrhea, insomnia, dyspepsia, anorexia, or leg cramps [6, 7].

Naturopathic therapy of AD uses herbal and nutritional intervention which have been shown to be as effective as prescription medications. Over 50 clinical trials have shown that ginkgo can be as effective in treating AD as medications, but without the side effects[8]. Ginkgo is believed to act as an anti-inflammatory, antioxidant, and it protects and strengthens nerve cells. Rare side effects reported with ginkgo use include stomach or intestinal upset, headaches, allergic skin reactions, and dizziness. When used with SSRIs it has been reported to reverse the sexual side effects caused by SSRIs [9, 10].

Asian ginseng has also been reported to increase memory, learning, and mental functioning, but should not be used by people on blood thinning medications or MAOIs[11, 12]. Sage, a herb that has been reported to have been used in traditional Chinese medicine, Ayurvedic medicine and European herbal medicine is believed to inhibit the production of acetylcholinesterase, an enzyme that is associated with the development of AD[13].

Nutritional interventions for AD uses vitamin E [14], B-complex [15], Choline [16], an amino acid, L-carnitine [17], and essential fatty acids, DHA [18]. All believed to supply the brain and nervous system essential nutrients to function properly and fight environmental toxins.

Anxiety

Anxiety disorders are the most common psychiatric disorder in children, and often foreshadows later mental illness such as depression [19]. Anxiety disorders are classified as panic disorders, agoraphobia, specific phobia, social phobia, obsessive compulsive disorder (OCD), posttraumatic stress disorder (PTSD), acute stress disorder and generalized anxiety disorder (GAD). Most anxiety disorders typically start during late adolescence and early adulthood [20].

Anxiety can be linked to physiological changes in the amygdala and hippocampus portions of the brain. Neurochemicals involved in these pathways include GABA, serotonin, and norepinephrine [21]. Other biochemical responses to anxiety and stress in the body involve the adrenal glands that produce adrenaline, cortisol, and CRF, which are overproduced during stress [22]. By applying a kindling model of behavior to biochemical changes in the brain it can be explained how subsequent less stimuli can elicit a greater response to anxiety and stress. As elevated levels of CRF are present in the brain, less stimuli is needed to achieve a greater response, causing increased anxiety and stress [23].

Environmental toxins may also cause biochemical reactions that increase the likelihood of stress. High copper levels have been linked to low blood levels of histamine, that have been associated with behavioral abnormalities [24]. Recent studies have also linked anxiety to faulty lactic acid metabolism. It has been observed that people that suffer panic attacks have high levels of lactic acid in their blood, as they are unable to convert lactate to harmless pryruvic acid [25].

Allopathic treatment of anxiety and stress disorders is with various neurochemical agents such as benzodiazepines that inhibit GABA receptors in the brain, but may have side effects of sedative or hypnotic effects, anticonvulsant actions, muscle relaxant effects, ataxia or amnesia. Propranolol, a β-blocker, is used for anxiety disorders and does not dim consciousness or produce drug dependence like benzodiazepines, however, it could cause fatigue, depression, liver and kidney impairment. Antihistamines are often prescribed for anxiety disorders due to their sedating effects, but they are not recommended for long term use and may cause drowsiness, dry mouth, twitches, tremors, and convulsions[26]. Antidepressants like TCAs, and SSRIs have been prescribed for anxiety disorders, but come with side effects ranging from mild (dry mouth, nausea, headaches) to severe (seizures, liver damage, heart problems, hypertension, strokes, death)[27].

Naturopathic treatment for anxiety uses herbal therapy and a number of relaxation therapies that are believed to be effective. A number of studies support American ginseng's use as a sedative herb. Ginsenosides in ginseng are believed to reduce stress by increasing the blood flow to the brain, improving concentration and mental performance. Side effects have been reported with excessive amounts of ginseng such as diarrhea, diminished libido, earaches, high blood pressure, insomnia, rashes, nosebleeds, and vomiting [28].

Another herb that has been studied for its effectiveness on anxiety and stress that has been used for centuries in the South Pacific, is kava. Kavalactones, the active ingredient in kava has a calming effect by elevating mood and increasing mental alertness. Like ginseng, side effects have been reported with overdoses[29]. Other therapeutic herbs used for relieving stress and anxiety include lavender, skullcap, valerian, chamomile, lemon balm, and passionflower [30].

Nutritional intervention is believed to alleviate anxiety and stress when a contributing cause may be nutrient deficiencies. Calcium and magnesium supplements will help lower lactate production.

Essential fatty acids such as ALA have been shown to be helpful in treating anxiety. Supplements of vitamins a, B-complex, C, E, pantothenic acid and minerals of calcium, potassium, and magnesium, all contribute to proper adrenal gland and nervous system function [31, 32, 33, 34, 35, 36].

Other alternatives relaxation therapies have been proven to be helpful in relieving stress and anxiety. Yoga has been found to be effective with OCD [37]. Studies have shown anxiety has been reduced using Transcendental Meditation, used for centuries in Ayurvedic medicine [38]. Meditation produces a state of mind called blanking out, which is a deep relaxation state. This state greatly reduces stress-related biochemicals such as adrenaline and cortisol, as well as decreasing blood pressure and heart rate. Devices such as a floatation tank have been used to achieve a blanking out state that has been shown to reduce stress and anxiety for days after use [39].

Aromatherapy uses essential oils to treat stress and anxiety. Relaxing bath oils or massage oils of clary sage, lavender, jasmine, melissa (lemon balm), neroli, marjoram, rose and ylang-ylang are reported to relieve stress [40, 41].

ADHD

Attention Deficit/Hyperactivity Disorder (ADHD) is considered one of the most common childhood neurobehavioral disorders of school-aged children, believed to effect between 4 to 12 percent of all children. The American Academy of Pediatrics (AAP) believes ADHD may be over diagnosed by physicians, and calls for stricter adherence to DSM-IV criteria before placing a child on psychostimulate medication [42].

Allopathic medicine appears to down play specific causes of ADHD, indicating it may be the result of several factors such as genetic, prenatal damage from teratogens, or postnatal damage such as in lead poisoning or head trauma [43]. Other theories include chemical imbalances such as faulty glucose metabolism, thyroid abnormalities or fatty acid deficiency [44]. Adverse reaction to sugar remains a controversial topic as a probable cause of ADHD.

In the 1970's Dr. Ben Feingold theorized that hyperactive children are sensitive to naturally occurring salicylates and phenolic compounds in found in foods after researching over 1,200 cases of hyperactive children. He showed that by eliminating salicylates, artificial colors, and artificial flavors from hyperactive children's diets there were significant improvements in their behavior [45]. Several studies since the 1970's support Dr. Feingold's research. Studies involving hundreds of ADHD children in the 1980's and 1990's report children being adversely affected by their diet, the worst offender being sugar [46, 47, 48].

Glucose levels (blood sugar) have been related to adrenaline levels in the blood particularly when there is faulty glucose metabolism causing an increase in adrenaline in the presence of sugar [45]. A thyroid dysfunction may be responsible for the altered glucose metabolism found in ADHD children. Thyroid dysfunction may be caused by synthetic chemicals like PCBs, phenols, thiols, excessive histamines, or a deficiency in EFAs [50].

Allopathic treatment of ADHD uses psychostimulates, the most prescribed medication for children over the past three decades being Ritalin (Methylphenidate hydrochloride). Ritalin is a central nervous system (CNS) stimulate that is believed to work for ADHD individuals by activating the brainstem arousal system which has an effect of decreasing motor restlessness, increasing attention span and concentration. Ritalin is a CNS stimulate that is in the same class of drugs as amphetamines and cocaine, and is believed to be as habit forming, and lead to physical and psychological dependence likes other drugs in this category. Newer CNS psychostimulates prescribed for ADHD like Concerta, Cylert, Dexedrine, Tofranil, Norpramin, and Adderall, all have side effects that can range from mild (anorexia, insomnia, irritability, nausea, depression, blurred vision, dry mouth, constipation, dizziness) to serious (high blood pressure, suppressed growth, liver damage and psychosis) [51, 52].

Alternative treatment for ADHD attempts to address the cause of the disorder. Dr. Fiengold pioneered the first naturopathic approach to treating ADHD through the process of an elimination diet. By eliminating all foods that contain natural and synthetic salicylates for four to six weeks behavior can be normalized. Once the ADHD behavior has diminished, foods items can slowly be reintroduced and monitored for their effect on the child's behavior [53].

Other than allergic reactions to specific foods or glucose (sugar), other researchers recommend nutritional intervention by correcting nutrient deficiencies that may be the cause of ADHD. Increasing protein in the diet increases serotonin levels in the brain, that can have a calming effect on children with hyperactivity, B-complex vitamins, with extra B_6 strengthens the nervous system. Vitamins A and C and minerals of calcium, magnesium, selenium and zinc, and essential fatty acids help protect against allergies and toxin damage [54, 55, 56, 57, 58, 59].

Recommended herbal therapy for ADHD includes the use of relaxing herbs such as kava kava, skullcap, ginseng, St. John's wort, passionflower, lavender, lemon balm and valerian [60, 61].

Depression

Depression is estimated to effect 1 out of 10 adults in their lifetime, or 17.5 million Americans in a every year. The illness results in an increased risk for medical illness and social disability [62]. Research indicates that depression is occurring at an earlier age, and more people are getting the illness than ever before [63].

In children, boys and girls get equally depressed, however, by adolescence the rate is 2:1 of females to males as it is in adults. Depression increases an individual's risk for substance abuse, suicidal behavior, and poor psychosocial function [64]. The DSM-IV-TR categorizes three main types of depressive disorder: Major Depressive Disorder (MDD), Dysthymic Disorder, and Depressive Disorder Not Otherwise Specified. MDD can be further classified as mild, moderate, severe without psychotic features, and severe with psychotic features [65].

The AMA states there are a number of theories as to the cause of depression, such as abnormal brain chemistry, abnormal levels of hormones or genetics. Three neurotransmitters have been linked to depression: dopamine, norepinephrine, and serotonin. These neurotransmitters effect the brain's pleasure centers, the hypothalamus and the limbic system. Endorphins are a type neuropeptides that have both neurotransmitter and hormonal qualities. It has been observed that people with depression have low levels of endorphins.

Depressed people also have low levels of an amino acid, GABA, that helps to control the flow of nerve impulses blocking the release of norepinephrine and dopamine. Hormonal irregularities are also linked to depression. The hypothalamus gland is responsible for regulating the pituitary gland that controls the secretion of hormones, and has been noted to use the same neurotransmitters involved in depression. High levels of cortisol, a hormone released by the adrenal gland during times of stress, has also been observed in people who are depressed. Researchers believe a number of genes may make an individual more susceptible to depression if inherited.

Environmental factors such as stressful situations, a loss or crisis, low self-esteem, high criticism, and feelings of lack of control can lead to depression [66, 67]. Depression can have several physical cause such as thyroid disease, diseases of the adrenal gland, complications from diabetes, infectious diseases such as mononucleosis, pneumonia, viral hepatitis, CFS, autoimmune disorders, degenerative disorders, cardiovascular disorders, or diseases of metabolism [68].

Nutrient deficiencies may lead to depression A lack of niacin and B-complex vitamins causes pellagra, of which depression is a symptom of. Depression can also be a symptom of anemia which is caused by an iron deficiency, or be related to deficiencies of sodium, magnesium, or zinc [69].

Many prescription medications can cause depression. Medications for high blood pressure, Parkinson's disease, NSAIDs used to relieve pain in arthritis, anticonvulsant medications used for seizure disorders, corticosteroid medications, used for allergies and inflammation and even oral contraceptives have been known to cause depression [70].

Allopathic treatment for depression usually involves antidepressant medication. Studies have shown that pharmacotherapy and psychotherapy works better than either treat alone, and that placebos used in clinical trails to be 50 percent as effective as antidepressants [71]. And, typically 20 to 35 percent of all patients fail to respond at all to antidepressant medication [72]. All antidepressant medications have side effects that can range from mild to severe. Antidepressants work by altering the brain's supply of neurotransmitters [73]. Tricyclic antidepressants have been used the longest for depression. They operate by blocking the reuptake of noreoinephrine or serotonin. Tricyclics often have side effects ranging from drowsiness, dry mouth, constipation, dizziness and heart palpitations to tremors, weight gain and sexual dysfunction [74].

MAOIs operate by preventing monoamine oxidase from breaking down neurotransmitters. Their side effects can include dizziness, changes in blood pressure, weight gain, insomnia, constipation, blurred vision, and reduced sexual functioning [75,76,77]. MAIOs also negatively impacts tyramine absorption and if foods are eaten containing tyramine severe side effects can ensue such as headaches, nausea, high blood pressure, stroke and even death [78].

SSRIs are newer antidepressants that function by increasing the brain's supply serotonin. They produce fewer side effects than MAIOs but may cause insomnia, nervousness, nausea, diarrhea, headaches and sexual dysfunction. Some atypical antidepressants can work by blocking the reuptake of dopamine or serotonin, others operate by increasing serotonin and norepinephrine. Side effects of atypicals can include weight gain, insomnia, headaches, nausea, tremors, increased blood pressure, sexual dysfunction, and seizures [78].

Lithium has been used to treat bipolar depression since the 1960's. researchers believe it may operate by blocking certain proteins that regulate neurotransmitters. Forty percent of people on lithium experience nausea, vomiting, diarrhea, stomachaches, headaches, acne, dry skin, or insomnia.

Anticonvulsants were developed to treat seizures, but also help bipolar depression. They function by blocking an amino acid, GABA, and in doing so the medication calms nerves. Side effects of anticonvulsants may include dizziness, drowsiness, headaches, double vision, nausea, diarrhea, skin rash, and possible liver damage [79, 80, 81].

Naturopathic treatment for depression uses herbal therapy, nutritional intervention, and other alternative remedies such as relaxation therapies. St. John's wort, a herb that has been used for more than 2,000 years for nervous disorders, has also been verified as a treatment for depression through several clinical studies over the past 20 years [82, 83].

St. John's wort is believed to work like a SSRI, by inhibiting serotonin, and inhibit a protein, Il-6, that has been shown to increase adrenal regulatory hormones [84]. Side effects of St. John's wort use has been reported as clinically insignificant, especially when comparing its use to prescription antidepressants. The FDA warns against St. John's wort use when using other prescription medications. There have been no deaths reported with the use of St. John's wort, however prescription antidepressants report 31 deaths per million prescriptions filled. St. John's wort is believed to reduce the effectiveness of a number of medications, therefore, it is recommended to discuss St. John's wort use with your physician if on any prescription medications [85, 86, 87].

A number of studies support the use of another herb, ginkgo for treatment of depression. Ginkgo has been used in Chinese medicine for over 5,000 years, and is believed to relieve depression by its ability to increase the supply of oxygen to the brain. Some reported side effects of ginkgo use include dizziness, upset stomach and rarely headache [88, 89].

Other herbs reported to have depression reducing effects are ginseng, kava and lavender. Ginseng is believed to relieve depression by improving blood flow to the brain, regulating hormones and increasing serotonin. Ginseng may cause insomnia, hypertension, diarrhea, and anxiety if taken in excess, and may interfere with hypertension or diabetic medication [90, 91, 92].

Kava has been reported to have been used as an antidepressant and sleep aid for over 3,000 years in the South Pacific. Researchers believe kava functions as an antidepressant by acting as a central nervous system sedative. Overdoses of kava have been reported to cause blurred vision, shortness of breath, skin irritation, and redden eyes. Kava may also interact negatively with other prescription medications for anxiety, depression and Parkinson's disease [93].

Lavender is considered an aromatic healing herb. It is used in soaps, perfumes, powders, sachets, teas, and essential oils. Used externally in aromatherapy, lavender's essential oil is used for relaxation, stimulation of the mind and to relieve depression [94]. Other essential oils believed to relieve depression include bergamot, clary sage, geranium, and neroli [95].

Nutritional intervention for depression uses supplements the body may be lacking. A popular treatment for depression in Europe, that first became available in the U.S. in 1999, is a combination of ATP and an amino acid, methionine, called S-adenosylmethionine (SAMe). SAMe is believed to work as an antidepressant by increasing the synthesis of serotonin and norepinephrine. Reported side effects of SAMe could include nausea and mania[96].

A poor diet and lack of essential nutrients are believed to contribute to depression. Junk foods depletes the body of B vitamins and calcium, important in neuron function, and places stress on the pancreas. Caffeine addiction creates thiamin deficiency and weakens the nervous system, too much meat can cause toxins and uric acid to accumulate in the blood. Alcohol depletes the body of nutrients and places strains the liver, pancreas, and kidneys. To counteract the effects of a deficient diet complex carbohydrates, protein from sources like fish or organically grown turkey, and supplements of vitamins A, B-complex, C, D, and minerals of calcium, magnesium, selenium, and zinc are recommended. Essential fatty acids also play important roles in nervous system function[97, 98, 99, 100].

Other alternative therapies such as acupuncture, exercise, yoga, light therapy, therapeutic massage, and biofeedback devices have been shown to reduce and alleviate depression[101, 102, 103].

Headaches and Migraines

It is estimated that 80 million Americans experience headaches, 50 million have experienced a migraine, and 28 million suffer from migraines regularly. Seventy percent of migraine suffers are women, and 30 percent of sufferers report getting a migraine before age ten[104].

Headaches are divided into four categories based on their symptoms and causes: tension headaches, the most common type, usually caused by muscle tension, organic headaches, usually caused by other illnesses like a tumor, and vascular headaches that can be either cluster headaches or migraines.

Cluster headaches are usually experienced by men (90 percent), can occur frequently in one day, and are usually on one side of the head. Migraines can be with or without aura (flashing lights or other sensory symptoms). Migraines usually progress in stages with a variety of physical symptoms such as tingling sensations, muscle stiffness, thirst, sensitivity to light and sound, irritability, cravings for sweets, and headache[105].

Headaches and migraines can be caused by a great number of factors. Organic causes include tumors, aneurysms, meningitis, head injuries, muscle and joint disorders, sleep disorders, and diseases[106, 107, 108, 109]. Tension headaches can be the result of stress[110]. Migraines are the result of blood vessels in the head constricting, and then dilating. There are several theories as to what sets off this process, that include changes in serotonin levels, magnesium levels in the body that regulate serotonin levels, hypothalamus dysfunction, hypoglycemia, food allergies, environmental toxins, and some prescription medications [110, 111, 112, 113, 114, 115, 116].

Allopathic treatment for headaches that are occasional recommends OTC pain relievers such as aspirin or acetaminophen that can be effective. However, if overused they can lead to stomach ulcers and even drug rebound headaches [117]. Prescription medications to treat migraines can be either abortive, to stop migraines, or prophylactic drugs that stops future ones from striking. Abortive drugs include corticosteroids, ergot derivatives, opioids or narcotics, NASIDS, triptans, and combination drugs. Side effects from these drugs can range from anxiety, insomnia, nausea, muscle cramps, dizziness, diarrhea, heartburn, to high blood pressure, heart problems and drug dependency. Prophylatic drugs for migraines include antidepressants, antiseizure medications, beta-blockers, calcium channel blockers, MAOIs, and botox. Side effects of these medications can include dry mouth, anxiety, insomnia, nausea, muscle cramps, dizziness, diarrhea, heartburn, weight loss, hair loss, sexual dysfunction, blurred vision, elevated blood pressure, heart problems, or psychotic problems [118, 119, 120].

Naturopathic treatment for headaches and migraines tries to determine the cause of the disorder first. A common cause of headaches and migraines are food allergies, and nutritional intervention would begin by eliminating potential offenders[121]. Nutritional intervention can also include supplements that increase blood flow such as magnesium, regulate hormones and blood cell production like riboflavin, and using herbs such as feverfew that inhibits inflammation [122, 123, 124, 125, 126].

Other nutritional intervention includes the use of cayenne pepper, quercetin, a bioflavonoid, niacin, vitamins A, B's, C, and E, and minerals of potassium, iron, iodine, and zinc, all responsible for proper nervous system function, fighting toxins and increasing oxygen in the blood [127, 128, 129]. EFAs are believed to help reduce the frequency of headaches by reducing inflammation [130].

Herbal therapy for headache and migraine relief include the use of valerian, that acts as a sedative and anti-spasmodic, chamomile and passionflower that relax and reduce pressure on blood vessels, ephedra, or ma-huang that has diuretic and anti-inflammatory effects, skullcap that is sedative, willow bark that is a natural aspirin, thyme, that has antiseptic and antispasmodic properties, doug quai, that has anti-inflammatory effects, and ginkgo, that increases cerebral circulation [131, 132, 133, 134, 135, 136].

Aromatherapy uses essential oils of herbs and plants to relieve headaches and migraines. Chamomile, lavender, marjoram, pennyroyal, peppermint, spearmint, rosemary and rose are used in diffusers or as massage oils for relief [137,138]. Other alternative therapies used to treat headaches and migraines include biofeedback training, acupuncture, exercise and special dental appliances [139, 140, 141, 142, 143, 144].

Bipolar Disorder

Bipolar Disorder or previously termed *manic-depressive* disorder is classified as a mood disorder. Mood disorders have been observed as far back as recorded history allows. The theories of the origins of mood disorders, and the controversy the continues today, can be credited to Krapelin (biological basis) and Freud (environmental reactions)[145]. The prevalence of major depression in ones lifetime can be as high as 18 percent. However, bipolar disorder affects only one percent of the population. Woman are at a greater risk for depression, with the age of onset in the late 20's, but bipolar disorder is equal among women and men with the average age of onset in the early 20's [146].

Bipolar Disorder is usually treated for the mania with antipsychotics, mood stabilizers or alternative agents. Lithium, lithium carbonate (*Eskalith),* Olanzapine (*Zyprexa),* or valproate acid (*Depakote*) are the drugs of choice for Bipolar Disorder. Lithium, valproate acid and carbamazepine (*Tegretol)* are usually treated for the mania of bipolar disorder, however, growing evidence suggests that these drugs may also reduce depression as well. The depression of Bipolar Disorder can be treated with SSRIs, TCAs, bupropion, or MAOIs [147].

Bipolar Disorder can be treated holistically by addressing symptoms of the mania and the depression. However, due to the severity of symptoms an individual may experience with Bipolar Disorder therapy should be prescribed by a naturopathic physician. To reduce the symptoms of mania, calming herbs such as American ginseng, Kava kava, Lavender, Skullcap/Virginian, Valerian, Passionflower, Chamomile, or Lemon balm can be used. Depression can be treated with St. John's wort, gingko or SAMe effectively [148].

Schizophrenia

Recent estimates that schizophrenia affects about 7 to 8 out of a 1,000 people of the population. Typically, symptoms begin in late adolescents or early adulthood. Men and woman share the frequency of the disorder, however, woman usually have a 5 year later onset of the disorder. The DSM-IV classifies schizophrenia as a psychotic disorder with a number of variations based on the symptoms. A common characteristic of schizophrenia, Schizophreniform

Disorder, Schizoaffective Disorder, and Brief Psychotic Disorder, are psychotic delusions, any prominent hallucinations, disorganized speech, and disorganized or catatonic behavior [149].

Antipsychotic medications are usually prescribed for Schizophrenia. Categories of medications that are used for Schizophrenia include: **Traditional agents;** (High-potency drugs) Fluphenazine (*Prolixin*), Haloperidol (*Haldol*), Thiothixene (*Navane*), Trifluoperazine (*Stelazine*), (Moderate-potency drugs) Loxapine (*Loxitane*), Molindone (*Moban*), Perphenazine (*Taractan*), (Low-potency drugs) Chlorpromazine (*Thorazine*), **Atypical Agents;** Clozapine (*Clozaril*), Olanzapine (*Zyprexa*), Quatrain (*Seroquel*), Risperidone (*Risperdal*). See *Table 7-3* for these medications and possible side-effects [150].

Dr. Carl Pfeiffer and the Brain Bio Center in New Jersey have studied mental disorders, and particularly Schizophrenia for over 50 years. He, and his Center have developed treatments for mental disorders based on nutritional deficiencies individuals may have. After treating thousands of patients diagnosed with Schizophrenia he determined there are five main "biotypes" based on their blood work: *Histapenia:* Low blood histamine with excess copper; *Histadelia:* High blood histamine with low copper; *Pyroluria:* A familial double deficiency of zinc and vitamin B_6; *Cerebral Allergy:* Includes wheat-gluten allergy and food additives; and *Nutritional Hypoglycemia* from faulty glucose metabolism. His therapy is based on the type of Schizophrenia and includes restrictive diets and supplements to counteract environmental toxins such as heavy metals [151].

Conclusions:

Allopathic (traditional western) treatment for mental disorders promotes the use of prescription medications to treat the symptoms of the disorder. With every medication studied there are reports of side effects. They can range from mild (dry mouth, nausea, diarrhea, muscle cramps, headaches) to severe (seizures, mania, psychosis, liver damage, heart problems, hypertension, strokes, death). Prevalence of side effects range widely with the medication, the length of time of use of the medication, and the individual taking the medication.

Although, allopathic physicians warn the public continually over the dangers of "untested" alternative treatments, they continually downplay the significant danger of prescription medications, as well as the poor safety record of the drugs. The American Medical Association estimates over 200,000 deaths per year from prescription medications, and another 2 million per year that require hospitalization for adverse side effects. Compared to the unproven alternative treatments, less than 20 deaths per year, there is little comparison as to which treatment is safer [152].

Allopathic physicians in America for the most part appear to be a product of the pharmaceutical revolution of the 20th century. As antibiotics and sulfa drugs were being developed and used in the mid 1900's interest in the newly discovered vitamins and what they are essential for in the body waned. As the pharmaceutical companies developed new drugs medical treatment emphasized curing the symptoms of the illness, as opposed to the illness, or the cause of the illness. Therein lies a major difference between the allopathic and naturopathic approaches. Allopathic physicians primarily treat symptoms of the disorder, whereas naturopathic treatment emphasizes determining the cause of the disorder, and cures the patient [153].

Naturopathic treatments appear to be controversial perhaps due to the variety of therapies offered. Should nutritional intervention, herbal treatment, aromatherapy, acupuncture, biofeedback or relaxation therapy be used remains a question that the novice often has difficulty answering. Most Americans become conditioned to rely solely on their "healthcare professional". And, if that professional is unknowledgeable about alternative treatments they will only recommend what they know, which are prescription medications. However, 70 to 90 percent of the world uses what the West calls alternative medicine [154].

The public is faced today with educating itself (or find a naturopathic physician) on treatment options when seeking other than allopathic treatment for their disorders. Today 40 percent of Americans opt for some sort of alternative medical treatment. Forty-eight percent of Americans take daily vitamin or mineral supplements, and an estimated $20 billion a year is spent out of their own pockets by Americans for alternative treatments. And, due to the continual demand for such options more and more information is surfacing.

Universities and medical schools are now offering courses in alternative treatments, and frequent articles appear in popular literature. Combining the modalities is called *Complementary* or *Integrative Medicine.* Americans are beginning to realize that "folk" remedies have survived for thousands of years because they work. Americans are learning what Europeans and Asians have known for a long time, that alternative therapies are effective, and they are without the side effects most prescription medications carry [155].

Naturopathic therapies for mental disorders can be a primary treatment rather than a secondary treatment. Nutritional intervention, herbal therapy, aromatherapy all lack side effects, unless substantially large amounts are taken. If side effects such as an allergic reaction does occur, discontinuation of that nutrient or herb will usually let the reaction subside [156].

Be open to what we might call the "unseen" world. The world that all religions are based on. That of believing you have an eternal soul, that your life has a purpose, and challenges in life are for a reason. This knowledge can do wonders to alleviate anxiety and depression, and make sense of all we go through in "classroom earth".

The "primary" treatment for mental disorders therefore, can be specific for the mental disorders discussed and general for overall mental health. Examples of specific treatment would be the use of ginkgo in Alzheimer's disease, American ginseng for anxiety disorders, nutritional interventions for ADHD, St. John's wort or SAMe for depression, feverfew, and nutritional supplementation for headaches and migraines.

Nutritional intervention may also cure a cause of a disorder that may be attributed to a poor diet, nutrient deficiencies, and an over abundance of toxins in the food supply and environment. Overall mental health has many commonalties, which is not surprising considering the following recommendations effect the health of the central nervous system:

Recommendations For Overall Mental Health:

- An organic diet of fresh vegetables, fruits, whole grains, with limited saturated fats. Try to eliminate all synthetic sugars and processed foods (packaged foods with additives and preservatives). Consume protein from cold water fish, 3 to 4 times per week (omega-3 EFA's) and eat lean meats like turkey or chicken breasts.

- Additional daily supplements of: multi-vitamin/mineral, B-complex (120-150 mg, per day), vitamin C (1,500 to 2,000 mg, per day), vitamin E (400 to 800 IUs, per day), Calcium (1,000 to 1,500 mg, per day), magnesium (300 to 500 mg, per day), selenium (75-100 mcg, per day), zinc (15 to 30 mg, per day).

- Additional essential fatty acids should be taken by eating cold water fish (salmon, tuna) or taking an Alpha-linolenic acid supplement daily.

- Restrict sugar, processed foods, alcohol, caffeine, and nicotine from the diet, they are all toxic to the nervous system.

In addition:

For Alzheimer's Disease:

- Ginkgo (120 to 240 mg, per day), Asian ginseng (150 to 250 mg, per day), DHA when not eating fish (300 mg, per day).

- Avoid consumption of alcohol (brain poison), caffeine (stimulate), nicotine (reduces oxygen supply to brain) and exposure to toxic metals like aluminum (cookware, antacids, deodorants) lead, mercury, copper, and iron.

- Exercise is often considered a "fountain of youth" as it increases the overall health of all body systems and helps the body get rid of toxins.

For Anxiety and Stress:

- Take American ginseng (1 gram per day) or Kava kava (60 to 120 mg, per day).

- If stress or anxiety is causing insomnia try Valerian an hour before bedtime (50 to 150 mg).

For ADHD:

- An evaluation with a naturopathic physician to determine if a food allergy exists and a dietary evaluation to determine if a nutrient deficiency exists.

- Eliminate all processed foods that contain artificial additives such as benzoic acid, BHA, BHT, MSG, butylene glycol, potassium bisulfate, potassium and sodium nitrate, sulfites, and tartrazines from the diet.

- Eliminate natural salicylates such as almonds, apples, apricots, berries, cherries, grapes, raisins, oranges, peaches, plums, prunes, strawberries, pickles, tomatoes, cucumbers and vinegar from the diet.

For Depression:

- Supplements of St. John's wort, SAMe, ginkgo, ginseng and kava all have been shown to be effective treatments for depression. Herbal interventions should not be used with prescription medications and patients should always check with their physicians before combining alternative treatments with prescription medications.

- Therapies such as aromatherapy, exercise, yoga, acupuncture, massage, and biofeedback may complement other therapies when used with nutritional intervention and supplementation, or herbal medicine in treating depression.

For Headaches and Migraines:

- Add feverfew daily of 50 mg in the a.m. and 50 mg in p.m. Increase during headache or migraine attacks to 500 to 1,000 mg.

- Unless cold water fish is eaten daily take EFA supplements (500 mg of evening primrose oil, and 1,000 mg of EPA fish oil daily).

- Rather than coffee drink decaffeinated chamomile, passionflower, ginger, lemon balm, linden, mint, or peppermint tea daily.

- Take a hot bath or get a therapeutic massage with essential oils of lavender, chamomile, peppermint, rosewood, spearmint, marjoram, or melissa.

- If feverfew does not appear to be effective after two months of daily supplements try willow bark, skullcap, doug quai or ginkgo supplements daily.

- If sufficient pain relief is not obtained from the above recommendations, go to an acupuncturist or try a clinic that specializes in biofeedback training.

For Bipolar Disorder:

- Eat an organic diet with foods such as whole grains, vegetables, fruits and fish. Drink only spring water.

- Eliminate processed foods from the diet (any with foods with chemical additives). Restrict sugar, and caffeine in the diet.

- Take a multi-vitamin/mineral daily with additional vitamin C (2-3,000 mg, per day) B-Complex (100 mg 2 times per day), vitamin E (400-800 IU's per day), calcium (1,200-1,500 mg, per day), magnesium (600-800 mg, per day) selenium (75-100 mcg, per day), zinc (30-40 mg, per day).

- Additional essential fatty acids should be taken by eating cold water fish (salmon, tuna) or taking an Alpha-linolenic acid supplement.

- Use aromatherapy at home by using scented oils, bath oils or soaps such as Lavender, Melissa or Rose. Try yoga or spend time each day in meditation.

- Get a therapeutic massage with essential oils such as Clary sage, Lavender, Melissa, Rose, or Ylang-Ylang.

For Schizophrenia:

- Consultation with a naturopathetic physician is recommended that can conduct blood, urine and allergy tests to determine the type of Schizophrenia (see chapter VII).

- Eliminate toxins from the environment and food supply by eating an organic diet with foods such as whole grains, vegetables, fruits and fish. Drink only spring water.

- Eliminate processed foods from the diet (any with foods with chemical additives). Eliminate any foods with additives such as food dyes and preservatives. Eliminate aspirin and foods with calculates. Eliminate sugar, alcohol, and caffeine in the diet.

- Follow specific vitamin and mineral supplementations above based on type of Schizophrenia.

- Use calming herbs such as American Ginseng, Kava kava, Valerian, Skullcap, Lavender, or Chamomile.

- Consultation with a Spiritual Healer.

For Spiritual Mental Health:

- When experiencing supernatural events like hearing voices or seeing energy consult with a lightworker (someone that is reputable, and that can themselves connect with spiritual energy).

- If experiencing physical pain that cannot be medically diagnosed seek out a spiritual healer.

- Read books like *Destiny of Souls* by Michael Newton, and *Messages from the Masters* by Brian Weiss, to gain an understanding of why we are here and why things happen in our lives.

And remember:

Treatment for medical conditions should always be conducted by your healthcare professional. According to the FDA only physicians are allowed to prescribe medications, and the suggestions in this book are for dietary changes and/or supplements only.

Future Implications:

Holistic mental health can be a viable option based on this research. As more and more studies and information comes to the public's eye they will learn of the benefits other "nontraditional" treatments for disorders such as Alzheimer's Disease, anxiety, stress, ADHD, depression, headaches and migraines, even Bipolar Disorder and Schizophrenia. When faced with the information "uncovered" in this book it is difficult not to develop a bias against prescription medications and favor alternative therapies.

The public is starting to realize that allopathic medicine treats the symptoms of the disorder, and not the cause. Primary allopathic treatment involves prescribing one medication after another (when the first does not work), and another to counteract the side effects of the first (or second) medication.

All prescription medications for mental disorders carry some risks of side effects ranging from mild to severe. Granted, not all users develop severe side effects all the time, however, there is the risk. And, considering how many people die and are hospitalized each year due to prescription drug use, the danger appears quite substantial. Considering the rise in use of alternative therapies such as herbs and nutritional supplementation, and the significant lack of document able evidence of the harm of such treatments (no significant side effects or deaths reported), there should be little question as to using it initially for the treatment of mental disorders. And, considering that the use nutritional intervention or herbal treatments dates back thousands of years, that translates to quite a safety record. In many cases treatments such as nutritional intervention does in fact uncover the cause of the disorder.

Not everything that makes individuals ill has a biological origin. There may be causes for mental and physical illness that goes beyond medical textbooks. New age literature can document centuries of what western medicine calls "supernatural" events and healings. And an understanding of other realms may lead to a better understanding of one's self

Why is there still such a controversy presently over treatment of mental disorders in this country? In Europe physicians do not hesitate to prescribe herbal treatments such as St. John's wort , ginkgo or kava more than they do prescription drugs. What is the difference between the European physicians and American physicians? Is it their medical training? Or, is it the traditions the culture might have in using more natural remedies? Is it that Americans pride themselves with developing innovations and new therapies for illness? Are the American doctors still caught up in the antibiotic revolution of the 20th century?

Or, is it the influence of the pharmaceutical companies on the American physicians? Pharmaceutical companies spend millions on advertising, lobbying and supplying physicians with free samples. Coupled with lack of training on alternative therapies, it is no doubt most American physicians only prescribe medications.

However, with the public's increasing demand for treatments without side effects American physicians need to educate themselves on viable alternatives. For the open-minded physicians there are the occasional articles in medical journals on various studies involving the benefits of nutrition of herbal supplements. But until physicians are required to take courses in nutrition and alternative therapies and to seek the cause of disorders, their knowledge of such practices will remain superficial and most likely be non-recommending.

The onus therefore, will still lie with the public to either educate themselves about naturopathic treatments (or seek out naturopathic physicians), and/or demand knowledgeable answers from their healthcare providers on such treatments. And, there appears to be substantial evidence available today in journal articles, texts, and clinical studies on alternative treatments for anyone seeking such information. In the future in the "west" Complementary and Integrative medicine will hopefully be the norm. Physicians will offer options for their patients that go beyond simply taking a drug. They will work with their patients to cure the individual and not just band-aide the symptoms. And perhaps (someday) even look further when a patient tells them of hearing or seeing things.

Suggested Further Reading:

For overall Health:

J.R.T. Davidson and K.M. Connor, *Herbs for the Mind,* (New York, NY: The Guilford Press, 2000).

A. Frances, and M. B. First, *Your Mental Health,* (New York, NY: Scribner. 1998).

J. S. McCombs, *Lifeforce, A Dynamic Plan for Health, Vitality, and Weight Loss,* (San Francisco, CA: Robert D. Reed Publishers. 2004).

T. Szasz, *The Myth of Mental Illness,* (New York, NY: Harper and Row, 1974).

L. Tenney, *Nutritional Guide A Comprehensive Reference for Better Health,* (Pleasant Grove, UT: Woodland Publishing. 1997).

B. Wiseman. *Psychiatry The Ultimate Betrayal,* (Los Angeles, CA: Freedom Publishing. 1995).

J. Kabot-Zinn. *Full Catastrophe Living,* (New York, NY: Dell Publishing, 1990).

For Alzheimer's Disease

M. Hutchison, *MegaBrain: New Tools and Techniques for Brain Growth and Mind Expansion,* (New York, NY: Ballantine Books, 1991).

J. Lokvig, & J.D. Becker, *Alzheimer's A to Z,* (Oakland, CA: New Haringer Publications. 2004).

J. Lombard, and C. Germano, *The Brain Wellness Plan,* (New York, NY: Kensington Books. 1997).

199

V.H. Mark, and J.P. Mark, *Brain Power: A Neurosurgeon's Complete Program to Maintain and Enhance Brain Fitness Throughout Your Life,* (Boston, MA: Houghton Mifflin Co. 1989).

S. Pedersen, *Ginkgo: Increase Intellect and Improve Circulation*, (New York, NY: Dorling Kindersley Publishing Co, 2000).

For Anxiety and Stress

R. J. Callahan. *Tapping The Healer Within.* (New York, NY: Contemporary Books. 2001).

W. Conkling. *Secrets of Ginseng.* (New York, NY: St. Martin's Paperbacks. 1999).

M. Siegel, and N. Burke. *Herbs for Health and Happiness,* (Alexandria, VA: Time Life Books. 1999).

For ADHD

P. R. Breggin. *Talking Back to Ritalin,* (Cambridge, MA: Perseus Publishing. 2001).

M. A. Block. *No More Ritalin: Treating ADHD Without Drugs,* (New York, NY: Kensington Publishing Corp. 1996)

B. F. Feingold. *Why Your Child Is Hyperactive.* (New York, NY: Random House, 1975).

F. Lawlis. *The ADD Answer.* (New York, NY: The Penguin Group. 2004).

D. S. Nambudripad. *Say Good-bye To ADD and ADHD.* (Buena park, CA: Delta Publishing Co. 1999).

D. B. Stein. *Ritalin Is Not The Answer.* (San Francisco, CA: Jossey-Bass Publishers, 1999).

For Depression

M. A. Brown. *When Your Body Gets The Blues.* (Emmaus, PA: Rodale Press, Inc. 2002).

C. Hobbs. *St. John's Wort The Mood Enhancing Herb.* (Loveland, CO: Interweave Press. 1997).

S. Grazi, and M. Costa. *SAMe: The European Arthritis and Depression Breakthrough.* (Rocklin, CA: Prima Publishing Co. 1999).

For Headaches and Migraines

S. Diamond, *Conquering Your Migraine*, (New York, NY: Simon & Schuster, 2001).

A. Mauskop, and B. Fox, *What Your Doctor May Not Tell You About Migraines*, (New York, NY: Warner Books, 2001).

For Bipolar Disorder/ Schizophrenia

C. C. Pfeiffer, *Nutrition and Mental Illness*, (Rochester, VT: Healing Arts Press. 1987).

For Spiritual Awakening & Healing

G. Braden, *The Divine Matrix, Bridging Time, Space, Miracles and Belief.* (Carsbad, CA: Hay House, Inc., 2007).

G. Braden, *Walking Between Worlds, The Science of Compassion*, (Bellevue, Radio Bookstore Press, 1997).

B. Brennan, *Hands of Light, A Guide to Healing Through the Human Energy Field*, (New York, NY: Bantam, Books, 1987).

P. Dubro, *Elegant Empowerment, The Evolution of Consciousness* (U.S.A: Platinum Publishing, 2002).

E. Holmes, *The Science of Mind, A Philosophy, A Faith, A Way of Life*, (New York, NY: Penguin Putnam Inc.,1938).

M. Newton, *Destiny of Souls*, (St. Paul, MN: Llewellyn Publications, 2004).

B. Marciniak, *Path of Empowerment, Pleiadian Wisdom for a World in Chaos*, (Novato, CA: New World Library, 2004).

D. Melchizedek, *Serpent of Light Beyond 2012*, (San Francisco, CA: Red Wheel/Weiser, 2007).

C. Myss, *Anatomy of Spirit, The Seven Stages of Power and Healing*, (New York, NY: Three Rivers Press, 1996).

E. Pearl, *The Reconnection: Heal Others, Heal Yourself*, (New York, NY:Hay House Publishing, 2003).

M. Sharp, *The Book of Life*, (Avatar Publications, 2003-2006).

M. Sharp, *The Dossier of Ascension*, (Avatar Publications, 2004-2006). www.michaelsharp.org

B. Weiss, *Messages From The Masters*, (New York, NY: Warner Books, 2000).

P. Yogananda, *Autobiography of a Yogi*, (New York, NY: Crystal Clarity Publishers, 1946).

END NOTES/ REFERENCES

CHAPTER I:
TRADITIONAL vs. ALTERNATIVE TREATMENT for MENTAL DISORDERS

[1] J.R.T. Davidson and K.M. Connor, *Herbs for the Mind,* (New York, NY: The Guilford Press, 2000),1-2.

[2] R. Epstein, *Our Mental Health,* (Psychology Today 32:2000) 44-48.

[3] National Mental Health Association, *Mental Disorders Are a Major Health Problem Worldwide, Says WHO,* (The Bell, The Newsletter of the National Mental Health Association, Dec. 2001)6.

[4] American Psychiatric Association, *The Diagnostic and Statistical Manual of Mental Disorders, 4th edition, Text Revision,* (Washington, DC: American Psychiatric Association, 2000) 156.

[5] V.H. Mark, and J.P. Mark, *Brain Power: A Neurosurgeon's Complete Program to Maintain and Enhance Brain Fitness Throughout Your Life,* (Boston, MA: Houghton Mifflin Co. 1989)12.

[6] D.S. Pine, ed. *Fluvoxamine for the Treatment of Anxiety Disorder in Children and Adolescents,* (New England Journal of Medicine. v. 344:17, 2001)1279-1285.

[7] J. T. Coyle, *Drug Treatment of Anxiety Disorders in Children,* (New England Journal of Medicine v.344:17, 2001)1326-1327.

[8] R. J. Goldberg *Depression in the Workplace: Economics and Interventions,* (Behavioral Healthcare Tomorrow v.10:6, 2001) 10-11.

[9] American Psychiatric Association, et al., *The Diagnostic and Statistical Manual of Mental Disorders, 4th edition, Text Revision,* 371-372.

[10] American Academy of Pediatrics (May1, 2000). *AAP Releases New Guidelines For Diagnosis of ADHD,* (Press release posted on the World Wide Web) AAP author. WWW:http://www.aap.org/advocacy/releases/mayadhd.htm. Retrieved June 1, 2000.

[11] A. Frances, and M. B. First, *Your Mental Health*, (New York, NY: Scribner. 1998)109.

[12] S. Diamond, *Conquering Your Migraine*, (New York, NY: Simon & Schuster, 2001) 2-3.

[13] A. Mauskop, and B. Fox, *What Your Doctor May Not Tell You About Migraines,* (New York, NY: Warner Books, 2001)6-7.

[14] R. Voelker,. *Migraine on the Rise*, (Journal of the American Medical Association. *v.* 282:20, 1999) 217.

[15] A. Seiegil, *The Dictionary of Disorders: How One Man Revolutionized Psychiatry.* (The New Yorker. 1/3/05)56-63.

[16] D.W. Sifton, ed. *The PDR Pocket Guide to Prescription Drugs*, (New York, NY: Simon & Schuster, Inc. 2002) 96,275,491.

[17] J. S. Maxmen, and N. G. Ward, *Psychotropic Drugs Fast Facts,* (New York, NY: W.W. Norton & Company, 1995) 255-257.

[18] Maxmen, et al., *Psychotropic Drugs Fast Facts,* 86-93.

[19] Sifton, ed. et al., *The PDR Pocket Guide to Prescription Drugs,* 27, 325, 378, 1092.

[20] Ibid, 68, 190,366, 599, 607,764, 1425.

[21] S. Pedersen, *Ginkgo: Increase Intellect and Improve Circulation*, (New York, NY: Dorling Kindersley Publishing Co, 2000) 6-7.

[22] M. Angell, and J. P. Kassirer, *Alternative Medicine the Risks of Untested and Unregulated Remedies,* (New England Journal of Medicine, v.330, 1998) 839-841.

[23] D. S. Nambudripad, *Say Good-bye To ADD and ADHD,* (Buena park, CA: Delta Publishing Co. 1999) 22-26.

[24] S. Althoff, P. N. Williams, D. Molvig, and L. Schuster, *A Guide to Alternative Medicine,* (Lincolnwood, IL: Publications International Ltd., 1997)88-89.

[25] W. Conkling, *Secrets of Ginkgo*, (New York, NY:St. Martin's Press, 1999) 32-35.

[26] S. Pedersen, *Kava: Relax Your Muscles & Mind*, (New York, NY: Dorling Kindersley Publishing Co., 2000)33-35.

[27] J. Carper. *Miracle Cures.* (New York, NY: Harper Collins Publishers. 1997)58-70.

[28] S. Pedersen. *Ginkgo: Increase Intellect and Improve Circulation.* (New York, NY: Dorling Kindersley Publishing Co. 2000)8-10.

[29] V. E. Tyler, *Herbal Hope for Alzheimer's, Cancer, and Prostrate Disease,* (*Prevention.* v53:3, 2001)105-106.

[30] Pedersen, et al., *Kava: Relax Your Muscles & Mind,* 4-7.

[31] H. M. Lyman, C. Fenger, H. W. Webster, and W. T. Belfield. *The New*

American Family Physician, (Chicago, IL:Reily & Britton Co., 1905)1090-1095.

[32] A. Hoffer, and M. Walker. *Orthomolecuar Nutrition, New Lifestyle for Super Good Health.* (New Canaan,CT:Keats Publishing,Inc. 1978)1-3, 12-13.

[33] J. D. Walker, *The Skinny On Supplements. (Healthcare Directions, v.3:6, 2002)*22-23.

[34] M. Angell, and J .P. Kassirer, *Alternative Medicine the Risks of Untested and Unregulated Remedies. (New England Journal of Medicine.* v.330, 1998)839-841.

[35] I. Burk, *The ABCs of OTCs, Herbals and Supplements, (Student Assistance Journal,* v.14:2, 2001)16-19.

[36] V. E. Tyler, *The Truth About FDA Approval, (Prevention* v.53:6, 2001)119-121.

[37] B. Goldberg, *The Science of Deceit, (Alternative Medicine* v. 46, 2002)12-15.

CHAPTER II:
Alzheimer's DISEASE

[1] American Psychiatric Association. ed. *Diagnostic and Statistical Manual of Mental Disorders-Fourth Edition-Text Revision,* (Washington, DC: APA. 2000) 154-158.

[2] K. S. Berger, *The Developing Person Through the Life Span.* (New York, NY: Worth Publishers.1998) 647-649.

[3] J. Cummings, *Alzheimer's Disease. (New England Journal of Medicine, v351, 2004).* 56-67.

[4] J. Lombard, and C. Germano, *The Brain Wellness Plan,* (New York, NY: Kensington Books. 1997)65.

[5] American Psychiatric Association. ed. et al., *Diagnostic and Statistical Manual of Mental Disorders-Fourth Edition-Text Revision,* 154-158.

[6] Ibid, 154-156.

[7] Berger, et al., *The Developing Person Through the Life Span.* 647-649.

[8] O. Colliot. *New Type of MRI Scan Spots Alzheimer's. (Radiology,July 2008; v248)* 194-201.

[9] C. C. Pfeiffer, *Nutrition and Mental Illness,* (Rochester, VT: Healing Arts Press. 1987)73-76.

[10] L. Tenney, *Nutritional Guide A Comprehensive Reference for Better Health,* (Pleasant Grove, UT: Woodland Publishing. 1997)115.

[11] J. S. Bland, *Genetic Nutritioneering*. (Los Angeles, CA: Keats Publishing, 1999)61-71.

[12] Lombard, et al., *The Brain Wellness Plan*, 57-81.

[13] American Psychiatric Association. ed. et al., *Diagnostic and Statistical Manual of Mental Disorders-Fourth Edition-Text Revision*, 154-158.

[14] J. Travis, *Enzyme Offers Promise of Alzheimer's Drugs*. (*Science News*. v156,1999)294.

[15] M. Hutchison, *MegaBrain: New Tools and Techniques for Brain Growth and Mind Expansion*, (New York, NY: Ballantine Books, 1991)128,306.

[16] Lombard, et al., *The Brain Wellness Plan*, 57-81.

[17] E. M. Reiman, R. J. Caselli, L. S. Yun, K. Chen, D. Bandy, S. Minoshima, S. N. Thibodeau, and D. Osborne. *Preclinical Evidence of Alzheimer's Disease in Persons Homozygous for the ∈ 4 Allele for Apolipoprotein E.* (*The New England Journal of Medicine*. v334:12, 1996)752-758.

[18] C. W. Henderson, *On-The-Job Lead Exposure Could Increase Risk*. (Medical Letter on the CDC & FDA. 2000)1.

[19] Lombard, et al. *The Brain Wellness Plan*, 57-81.

[20] U. Dreses-Werringloer. *New Alzheimer's Gene. (Cell, v133, 6/27/08)1149-1161*.

[21] Mayo Clinic ed., *Successful Aging*, (Rochester, MN: Mayo Foundation. 2000)3-4.

[22] M. Moran, *Estrogen May Delay Dementia*. (*American Medical News*. v43,2000)21.

[23] R. Mayeux, and M. Sano, *Treatment of Alzheimer's Disease*. (*The New England Journal of Medicine*. v22,1999)167.

[24] L. Murray, ed., *The PDR Pocket Guide to Prescription Drugs*, (New York, NY: Simon & Schuster, Inc. 2008) 96, 275, 491.

[25] R. Voelker., *Promising Alzheimer Drug*. (*JAMA, Journal of the American Medical Association*. v283, 2000)2379.

[26] Henderson, et al., *On-The-Job Lead Exposure Could Increase Risk*. 1.

[27] H. W. Griffith, *Complete Guide to Prescription & Nonprescription Drugs*. (New York, NY: the Berkley Publishing Group. 2004).

[28] Moran, et al., *Estrogen May Delay Dementia*. 21.

[29] E. McGeer, *Soothing the Inflamed Brain: Anti-inflammatories May be the First Drugs to Halt the Progression of Alzheimer's*. (*Scientific America*. v282, 2000)24.

[30] B. Loecher, *Vaccine for Alzheimer's Possible*. (*Prevention*. v51, 1999)169.

[31] A. Atri. *Alzheimer's Disease and Associate Disorders. (Online edition: Department of Neurology and Massachusetts Alzheimer's Disease Research*

Center, Massachusetts General Hospital Harvard Medical School, Boston, MA. July/Sept. 2008).

32 T. Laughren. *Antipsychotics for Dementia Up Death Risk. (FDA News Release: July 16, 2008).*

33 S. Altshul, *Get Ginkgo: The Brain Tune-Up Herb. (Prevention.* v52, 2000) 50.

34 P. A. Balch, *Prescription For Herbal Healing,* (New York, NY: Avery Books. 2002)190-191.

35 J. R. T. Davidson, and K. M. Connor. *Herbs for the Mind.* (New York, NY: The Guilford Press. 2000)146-166.

36 Altshul, et al., *Get Ginkgo: The Brain Tune-Up Herb.* 50.

37 J. Carper. *Miracle Cures.* (New York, NY: Harper Collins Publishers. 1997)58-70.

38 Davidson, et al., *Herbs for the Mind.* 159-162.

39 W. Conking. *Secrets of Ginkgo.* (New York, NY: St. Martin's Press, 1999)33-39.

40 S. Pedersen. *Ginkgo: Increase Intellect and Improve Circulation.* (New York, NY: Dorling Kindersley Publishing Co. 2000)30-37.

41 A. B. Waltman. *A Guide to Natural Health. (Psychology Today.* v 33, 2000) 37.

42 Carper, et al., *Miracle Cures.* 58-70.

43 Davidson. et al., *Herbs for the Mind.* 159-162.

44 S. W. Lininger. *A-Z Guide to Drug-Herb-Vitamin Interactions,* (Roseville, CA: Prima Publishing. 1999)95,98.

45 L.G. Miller. *Selected Clinical Consideration Focusing on Known or Potential Drug-Herb Interactions,* (Journal of The American Medical Association. v158:20, 1998) 125-1127.

46 Balch. et al., *Prescription For Herbal Healing,* 190-191.

47 Conking. et al., *Secrets of Ginkgo.* 33-39.

48 Lininger et al., *A-Z Guide to Drug-Herb-Vitamin Interactions,* 95,98.

49 Davidson. et al., *Herbs for the Mind.* 159-162.

50 V. E. Tyler, *Herbal Hope for Alzheimer's, Cancer, and Prostrate Disease,* (*Prevention.* v53:3, 2001)105-106.

51 Environmental Nutrition. Ed. *Vitamin E May Slow Alzheimer's Decline.* v. 20 (1997)8.

52 L. Chang. *Vitamin E May Up Alzheimer's Survival. (News Release: American Academy of Neurology 60th Annual Conference, Chicago. April 12-19, 2008).*

53 R. Lethem, and M. Orrell. *Antioxidants and Dementia,* (The Lancet. v349, 1997) 1189.

54 Pfeiffer, et al., *Nutrition and Mental Illness,* 73-76.

55 E. Mindell, *Earl Mindell's Food as Medicine*, (New York, NY: Simon & Schuster. 1994)68.

56 L. Tenney, *Nutritional Guide A Comprehensive Reference for Better Health*, (Pleasant Grove, UT: Woodland Publishing. 1997)115.

57 L. Parch, *Brain Boosters, (Natural Health*, v35:5, 2005)45-53.

58 Ma, Q. *Fish Oil Prevents Alzheimer's Plaques. (Journal of Neuroscience, v27. December 26, 2007.) 14299-14307.*

59 Fiala, M. *Curry Spice May Counter Alzheimer's. (Proceedings of the National Academy of Sciences: online edition. July 2007).*

60 L. Parch, *Brain Boosters, (Natural Health*, v35:5, 2005) 45-53.

61 L. Tenney, *Nutritional Guide A Comprehensive Reference for Better Health*, (Pleasant Grove, UT: Woodland Publishing. 1997)115.115.

62 Lombard, et al., *The Brain Wellness Plan*, 57-81.

63 Ibid, 57-81.

64 Ibid, 57-81

65 J. Lokvig, & J.D. Becker, *Alzheimer's A to Z*, (Oakland, CA: New Haringer Publications. 2004) 4-90.

66 R.S. Doody. *Dimebon Shines as Alzheimer's Therapy. (The Lancet. v372. July 19, 2008)* 207-215.

67 H. Qiny. *Valproic Acid May Treat Alzheimer's. (The Journal of Experimental Medicine. October 27, 2008).*

68 K. Green. *Form of B3 May Help Alzheimer's. (Journal of Neuroscience. November 5, 2008).*

69 R.S. Doody. *Dimebon Shines as Alzheimer's Therapy. (The Lancet. v372. July 19, 2008)* 207-215.

70 Ibid, 207-215.

71 Ibid, 207-215.

CHAPTER III:
ANXIETY & STRESS DISORDERS

1 L. Iannotti. *The United States of Anxiety. (WebMD online article: January 16, 2009).*

2 D. S. Pine, ed. *Fluvoxamine for the Treatment of Anxiety Disorder in Children and Adolescents. (New England Journal of Medicine.* v.344:17, 2001)1279-1285.

3 C. T. Coyle. *Drug Treatment of Anxiety Disorders in Children. (New England Journal of Medicine* v.344:17, 2001)1326-1327.

4 American Psychiatric Association. ed. *Diagnostic and Statistical Manual of*

Mental Disorders-Fourth Edition-Text Revision, (Washington, DC: APA. 2000) 429-470.

[5] G. A. Bernstein, C. M. Borchardt, and A. R. Perwin. *Anxiety Disorders in Children and Adolescents A Review of the Past 10 Years. (Journal of American Academy of Child and Adolescent Psychiatry.* v.35:9, 1996)1110-1119.

[6] M. Murray, and J. Pizzorno. *Encyclopedia of Natural Medicine.* (Rocklin, CA: Prima Publishing. 1991)91-99.

[7] R. Epstein. *Stress Busters. (Psychology Today.* v.33:2, 2000) 30-36.

[8] American Psychiatric Association. ed. et al., *Diagnostic and Statistical Manual of Mental Disorders-Fourth Edition-Text Revision,* 429-430.

[9] D. R. Weinberger. *Anxiety at the Frontier of Molecular Medicine. (New England Journal of Medicine.* v.3442001)1247-1249.

[10] Ibid, 1247-1249.

[11] P. D. Kramer, *Listening to Prozac.* (New York, NY: Penguin Books.1994)101.

[12] Ibid, 101.

[13] C. C. Pfeiffer. *Nutrition and Mental Illness,* (Rochester, VT: Healing Arts Press. 1987)26-28.

[14] P. A. Balch. *Prescription For Herbal Healing,* (New York, NY: Avery Books. 2002)190-191.

[15] Coyle, et al., *Drug Treatment of Anxiety Disorders in Children.* 1326-1327.

[16] N. L. Keltner, D.G. Folks. *Psychotropic Drugs - Third Edition.* (St. Louis,MI. Mosby, Inc. 2001) 127-165.

[17] Ibid, 127-135.

[18] J. S. Maxmen, and N.G. Ward. *Psychotropic Drugs Fast Facts,* (New York, NY: W.W. Norton & Company. 1995)255-309.

[19] L. Murray, ed. *The PDR Pocket Guide to Prescription Drugs,* (New York, NY: Simon & Schuster, Inc. 2008) 96, 275, 491.

[20] D. R. Weinberger. *Anxiety at the Frontier of Molecular Medicine. (New England Journal of Medicine.* v.3442001)1247-1249.

[21] J. S. Maxmen, and N.G. Ward. *Psychotropic Drugs Fast Facts,* (New York, NY: W.W. Norton & Company. 1995)255-309.

[22] Murray, ed. et al., *The PDR Pocket Guide to Prescription Drugs.* 96, 275, 491.

[23] Maxmen, et al., *Psychotropic Drugs Fast Facts,* 255-309.

[24] Murray, ed. et al., *The PDR Pocket Guide to Prescription Drugs.* 96, 275, 491.

[25] Keltner, et al., *Psychotropic Drugs -Third Edition.* 127.

[26] Maxmen, et al., *Psychotropic Drugs Fast Facts,* 255-309.

[27] Murray, ed. et al., *The PDR Pocket Guide to Prescription Drugs.* 96, 275, 491.

²⁸ W. Z. Potter, M. V. Rudorfer, and H. Manji. *The Pharmacological Treatment of Depression. (New England Journal of Medicine.* v.325:9, 1991) 633-641.

²⁹ Murray, ed. et al., *The PDR Pocket Guide to Prescription Drugs.* 96, 275, 491.

³⁰ Coyle, et al., *Drug Treatment of Anxiety Disorders in Children.* 1326-1327.

³¹ M. Hiti. *Antipsychotic Drug May Ease Anxiety. (News release: European College of Neuropsychopharmacology, Barcelona, Spain. Aug. 30-Sept. 3, 2008).*

³² Coyle, et al., *Drug Treatment of Anxiety Disorders in Children.* 1326-1327.

³³ M. Angell, and J. P. Kassirer. *Alternative Medicine the Risks of Untested and Unregulated Remedies. (New England Journal of Medicine.* v.330, 1998) 839-841.

³⁴ E. Isaacs. *Fluvoxamine for the Treatment of Anxiety Disorder in Children and Adolescents. (New England Journal of Medicine.* v.345:6, 2001)466-467.

³⁵ W. Conkling. *Secrets of Ginseng.* (New York, NY: St. Martin's Paperbacks. 1999)58-60.

³⁶ Ibid, 58-60.

³⁷ Ibid, 58-60.

³⁸ Ibid, 58-60.

³⁹ S. W. Lininger. *A-Z Guide to Drug-Herb-Vitamin Interactions*, (Roseville, CA: Prima Publishing. 1999)95,98.

⁴⁰ M. Siegel, and N. Burke. *Herbs for Health and Happiness,* (Alexandria, VA: Time Life Books. 1999)95-96.

⁴¹ D. G. Williams. *Alternatives For The Health Conscious Individual: The Happiness Herb.* (Potomac, MD: Phillips Health. 2001)1-2.

⁴² Siegel, et al., *Herbs for Health and Happiness,* 95-96.

⁴³ Ibid, 95-96.

⁴⁴ R. Somerville. ed. *The Drug and Natural Medicine Advisor.* (Richmond, VI: Time-Life Books. 1997)697-698.

⁴⁵ Siegel, et al., *Herbs for Health and Happiness,* 93-96.

⁴⁶ Somerville. ed. et al.,. *The Drug and Natural Medicine Advisor.* 433.

⁴⁷ H. M. Lyman, C. Fenger, H. W. Jones, and W. T. Belfield. *The New American Family Physician.* (Chicago, Il: Reilly & Britton Co. 1905)340.

⁴⁸ Siegel, et al., *Herbs for Health and Happiness,* 93-96.

⁴⁹ Somerville. ed. et al., *The Drug and Natural Medicine Advisor.* 195-196.

⁵⁰ Siegel, et al., *Herbs for Health and Happiness,* 93-96.

⁵¹ Somerville. ed. et al., *The Drug and Natural Medicine Advisor.* 461.

⁵² Siegel, et al., *Herbs for Health and Happiness,* 93-96.

⁵³ S. A. O'Donnell. *Healing Herbs: 200 Natural Cures That Work.* (Emmaus, PA: Rodale Press, Inc. 1999)71-81.

⁵⁴ Somerville. ed. et al., *The Drug and Natural Medicine Advisor.* 580.

55 Siegel, et al., *Herbs for Health and Happiness,* 93-96.

56 Balch, et al., *Prescription For Herbal Healing,* 190-191.

57 M. D. Eades. *The Doctor's Complete Guide To Vitamins and Minerals.* (New York, NY: Dell Publishing. 1994)464-466.

58 E. M. Haas. *Staying Healthy with Nutrition.* (Berkeley, CA: Celestial Arts. 1992)740-741.

59 E. Mindell. *Earl Mindell's Food as Medicine,* (New York, NY: Simon & Schuster. 1994) 238-240.

60 M. Murray, and J. Pizzorno. *Encyclopedia of Natural Medicine.* (Rocklin, CA: Prima Publishing. 1991)91-99.

61 P. Pitchford. *Healing With Whole Foods: Oriental Traditions and Modern Nutrition.* (Berkeley, CA: North Atlantic Books. 1993)179.

62 R. Reinscheid. *New Insights on Anxiety, Sleep Disorders. (Neuron. V43. August 19, 2004).*

63 L. Tenney. *Nutritional Guide A Comprehensive Reference for Better Health,* (Pleasant Grove, UT: Woodland Publishing. 1997)115.

64 Balch, et al., *Prescription For Herbal Healing,* 190-191.

62 D. Bromage. ed. *Winter Blues.* (Aromatherapy, Essential Oils For Mind and Body. v1:5, 2002)18-20.

65 D. Corydon Hammond. *Handbook of Hypnotic Suggestions and Metaphors.* (New York, N: W Norton and Co., 1990)4-6.

66 R. G. Meyer. *Practical Clinical Hypnosis,* (New York, NY: Lexington Books. 1992) 1-7.

67 Althoff, P. N. Williams, D. Molvig, and L. Schuster. *A Guide to Alternative Medicine,* (Lincolnwood, IL: Publications International Ltd., 1997)31-34.

68 M. Hutchison. *MegaBrain: New Tools and Techniques for Brain Growth and Mind Expansion,* (New York, NY: Ballantine Books, 1991)270-273.

69 M. Evans. *The Complete Guide to Natural Remedies,* (New York, NY: Lorenz Books, 1999)91-101.

70 J. Kabot-Zinn. *Full Catastrophe Living,* (New York, NY: Dell Publishing, 1990)1-14.

71 M. Lavabre. *Aromatherapy Workbook,* (Rochester, VT: Healing Arts Press, 1990)77,82,85,88.

72 Balch, et al., *Prescription For Herbal Healing,* 190-191.

73 Althoff, et al., *A Guide to Alternative Medicine,* 31-34.

74 Ibid, 31-34.

CHAPTER IV:
Attention-Deficit/Hyperactivity Disorder

1. American Academy of Pediatrics (2000, May1). AAP Releases New Guidelines For Diagnosis of ADHD. (Press release posted on the World Wide Web) AAP author. Retrieved June 1, 2000 ,WWW:http://www.aap.org/advocacy/releases/mayadhd.htm.

2. S. Boyles. *Experts Revisit Food Additives and ADHD. (WebMD online: May 22, 2008).*

3. A. Frances, and M. B. First. *Your Mental Health.* (New York, NY: Scribner. 1998)11-21.

4. M. Gordan. *Compare and Contrast. (Journal of Learning Disabilities.* 31,1998)592-594.

5. I. A. Hyman, A. Wojtowicz, K. D. Lee, E. Haffner, C. A. Fiorello, J. J. Storlazzi, and J. Rosenfeld. *School-Based Methylphenidate Placebo Protocols: Methodological and Practical Issues. (Journal of Learning Disabilities.* 31, 1998) 581-592.

6. American Psychiatric Association. ed. *Diagnostic and Statistical Manual of Mental Disorders-Fourth Edition-Text Revision,* (Washington, DC: APA. 2000) 85-93.

7. Ibid, 85-93.

8. American Academy of Pediatrics. et al., *AAP Releases New Guidelines or Diagnosis of ADHD.* WWW.

9. Ibid, WWW.

10. J. B. Hale, J. B. Hoeppner, M. B. DeWitt, D. L. Coury, D. G. Ritacco, and B. Trommer. *Evaluating Medication Response in ADHD: Cognitive, Behavioral, and Single-Subject Methodology. (Journal of Learning Disabilities* 31, 1998)595-607.

11. M. Gordan. *Compare and Contrast. (Journal of Learning Disabilities.* 31, 1998)592-594.

12. L. Tenney, et al., *Nutritional Guide A Comprehensive Reference for Better Health,* 273-275.

13. S. Weintraub. *Natural Treatments for ADD and Hyperactivity,* (Pleasant Grove, UT: Woodland Publishing, 1997)121-128.

14. National Association of School Psychologist ed. *Best Practices in School Psychology.* (Washington, DC: NASP. 1995)817-830.

15. Ibid, 817-830.

16. K. S. Berger, *The Developing Person Through the Life Span.* (New York, NY: Worth Publishers,1998)318-321.

17 R. Barkley. *The Scientific American Book of the Brain; Attention-Deficit Hyperactivity Disorder.* (New York, NY: The Lyons Press 1999)101-111.

18 J. Lombard, and C. Germano. *The Brain Wellness Plan*, (New York, NY: Kensington Books. 1997)151-173.

19 P. Shaw. *New Clues on Causes of ADHD. (Archives of General Psychiatry. v 64. August 2007)* 921-931.

20 D. B. Stein. *Ritalin Is Not The Answer.* (San Francisco, CA: Jossey-Bass Publishers, 1999)1-16.

21 M. Bricklin. *The Practical Encyclopedia of Natural Healing.* (Emmaus, PE: Rodale Press, 1983)101.

22 L. Murray, ed. *The PDR Pocket Guide to Prescription Drugs*, (New York, NY: Simon & Schuster, Inc. 2008) 27, 325, 378, 1092.

23 S. Nambudripad. *Say Good-bye To ADD and ADHD.* (Buena park, CA: Delta Publishing Co. 1999)76-77.

24 Lombard, et al., *The Brain Wellness Plan.* 158-161.

25 M. A. Block. *No More Ritalin: Treating ADHD Without Drugs,* (New York, NY: Kensington Publishing Corp. 1996)74-79.

26 I. Rosenfeld. *Doctor What Should I Eat?* (New York, NY: Random House. 1995)11-21.

27 American Academy of Pediatrics. et al., AAP Releases New Guidelines For Diagnosis of ADHD.

28 Lombard, et al., *The Brain Wellness Plan.* 158-161.

29 B. F. Feingold. *Why Your Child Is Hyperactive.* (New York, NY: Random House, 1975)15-18.

30 Weintraub, et al., *Natural Treatments for ADD and Hyperactivity*, 121-128.

31 Ibid, 121-128.

32 Weintraub, et al., *Natural Treatments for ADD and Hyperactivity*, 121-128.

33 Lombard, et al., *The Brain Wellness Plan.* 158-161. M. Salaman. *Foods That Heal.* (Menlo Park, CA: Statford Pub. 1989)98-101.

34 A. Kemp. *Research Suggests Limiting Food additive in Diet May Help Kids with ADHD. (BMJ, v336. May 24, 2008)*1144.

35 P. R. Breggin. *Talking Back to Ritalin,* (Cambridge, MA: Perseus Publishing. 2001)4-33.

36 Stein. *Ritalin Is Not The Answer.* (San Francisco, CA: Jossey-Bass Publishers, 1999)1-16.

37 N. L. Keltner, D.G. Folks. *Psychotropic Drugs - Third Edition.* (St. Louis, MI. Mosby, Inc. 2001)470-474,498-500.

38 J. S. Maxmen, and N.G. Ward. *Psychotropic Drugs Fast Facts,* (New York, NY: W.W. Norton & Company. 1995)351-364.

39 Murray, ed. et al., *The PDR Pocket Guide to Prescription Drugs*,27, 325, 378, 1092.

40 J.M. Swanson. *Do ADHD Drugs Stunt Kids Growth? (Journal of the American Academy of Child and Adolescent Psychiatry. v46. August 2007)*1014-1026.

41 H. R. Manasse Jr. *ADHD Drugs and CV Outcomes. (FDA Drug Safety and Risk Management Advisory Committee, Feb.9 2006).*

42 FDA Pediatric Advisory Committee Meeting, March 22, 2006.

43 American Heart Association Scientific Statement, April 21, 2008, Circulation Online Edition.

44 FDA News Release: Alert for Healthcare Professionals: Pemoline Tablets and Chewable Tablets (Marked as Cylert). October 25, 2005.

45 A.D. Mosholder. *FDA Examines Incidence of Psychotic Symptoms in Children Taking ADHD Medications. (Pediatrics. V123. February, 2009)*611-616.

46 B.S.G. Molina. *ADHD at 6, Alcoholic at 16? (Alcoholism: Clinical and Experimental Research. V31. April, 2007).*

47 Block, et al., *No More Ritalin: Treating ADHD Without Drugs*, 74-79.

48 Alternative Medicine Review. 2003 Aug; 8(3):319-30.

49 F. Lawlis. *The ADD Answer.* (New York, NY: The Penguin Group. 2004)109 137.

50 M. Bricklin. *The Practical Encyclopedia of Natural Healing.* (Emmaus, PE: Rodale Press, 1983)101.

51 C. C. Pfeiffer. *Nutrition and Mental Illness,* (Rochester, VT: Healing Arts Press. 1987)98-99.

52 Weintraub, et al., *Natural Treatments for ADD and Hyperactivity*, 121-128.

53 E. Mindell. *Earl Mindell's Food as Medicine,* (New York, NY: Simon & Schuster. 1994)238-240.

54 Block, et al., *No More Ritalin: Treating ADHD Without Drugs*, 74-79.

55 Lombard, et al., *The Brain Wellness Plan.* 158-161.

56 Tenney, et al., *Nutritional Guide A Comprehensive Reference for Better Health,* 273-275.

57 Nambudripad, et al., *Say Good-bye To ADD and ADHD.* 76-77.

58 Weintraub, et al., *Natural Treatments for ADD and Hyperactivity*, 121-128.

59 Tenney, et al., *Nutritional Guide A Comprehensive Reference for Better Health,* 273-275.

60 M. Salaman. *Foods That Heal.* (Menlo Park, CA: Statford Pub. 1989)101-121.

61 F. Lawlis. *The ADD Answer.* (New York, NY: The Penguin Group. 2004)109 137.

CHAPTER V:
DEPRESSION

1 R. J. Goldberg, *Depression in the Workplace: Economics and Interventions*, (Behavioral Healthcare Tomorrow 10:6, 2001) 10-11.

2 American Medical Association, ed. *Essential Guide To Depression.* (New York, NY: Pocket Books, 1998).

3 B. Birmaher, N. Ryan, D.E. Willianson, D.A. Brent, J. Kaufman, R.E. Dahl, J. Perel, B. Nelson. *Childhood and Adolescent Depression: A Review of the Past 10 Years.* (Journal of the American Academy of Child and Adolescent Psychiatry 35:11, 1996)1427-1428.

4 D. Malone . *CDC: 1 in 20 Americans Depressed. (NCHS Data Brief: Depression in the United States Household Population, 2005-2006. Sept. 2008).*

5 Birmaher, et al., *Childhood and Adolescent Depression: A Review of the Past 10 Years.*1427-1428.

6 American Psychiatric Association. ed. *Diagnostic and Statistical Manual of Mental Disorders-Fourth Edition-Text Revision,* (Washington, DC: APA. 2000)369-380.

7 Ibid, 369-380.

8 Birmaher, et al., *Childhood and Adolescent Depression: A Review of the Past 10 Years.*1427-1428.

9 American Medical Association, ed. et al., *Essential Guide To Depression.*62-68.

10 Ibid, 62-68.

11 Ibid, 62-68.

12 Ibid, 62-68.

13 Ibid, 64-68.

14 American Medical Association, ed. et al., *Essential Guide To Depression.*68-70.

15 Ibid, 68-70.

16 American Medical Association, ed. et al., *Essential Guide To Depression.*76-78.

17 Ibid, 76-78.

18 American Medical Association, ed. et al., *Essential Guide To Depression.*83-86.

19 Ibid, 83-86.

20 Birmaher, et al., *Childhood and Adolescent Depression: A Review of the Past 10 Years.*1427-1428.

[21] American Medical Association, ed. et al., *Essential Guide To Depression* 100-102.

[22] Ibid, 102-103.

[23] Ibid, 108-109.

[24] Ibid, 104-105.

[25] Ibid, 105-106.

[26] Ibid, 106-107.

[27] Ibid, 107-108.

[28] Ibid, 108-110.

[29] Ibid, 188-189.

[30] Ibid, 188-189.

[31] W.J.G. Hoogendijk. *Many Depressed Older Adults Lack Vitamin D. (Archives of General Psychiatry. V 65, May 2008)* 508-512.

[32] L. Tenney. *Nutritional Guide A Comprehensive Reference for Better Health,* (Pleasant Grove, UT: Woodland Publishing. 1997)165-166.

[33] C. C. Pfeiffer. *Nutrition and Mental Illness,* (Rochester, VT: Healing Arts Press. 1987)26-28.

[34] American Medical Association, ed. et al., *Essential Guide To Depression.*152-154.

[35] J. S. Maxmen, and N.G. Ward. *Psychotropic Drugs Fast Facts,* (New York, NY: W.W. Norton & Company. 1995)351-364.

[36] L. Murray, ed. *The PDR Pocket Guide to Prescription Drugs,* (New York, NY: Simon & Schuster, Inc. 2008)241, 373, 443, 449, 816, 867, 908, 920, 1036, 1060, 1133, 1262, 1262, 1374, 1421.

[37] American Medical Association, ed. et al., *Essential Guide To Depression.*154-156.

[38] Maxmen, et al., *Psychotropic Drugs Fast Facts,* 351-364.

[39] Murray, ed. et al., *The PDR Pocket Guide to Prescription Drugs,* 241,373, 443, 449, 816, 867, 908, 920, 1036, 1060, 1133, 1262, 1262, 1374, 1421.

[40] Maxmen, et al., *Psychotropic Drugs Fast Facts,* 351-364.

[41] Murray, ed. et al., *The PDR Pocket Guide to Prescription Drugs,* 241, 373, 443, 449, 816, 867, 908, 920, 1036, 1060, 1133, 1262, 1262, 1374, 1421.

[42] American Medical Association, ed. et al., *Essential Guide To Depression.*156-160.

[43] Ibid, 156-160.

[44] Maxmen, et al., *Psychotropic Drugs Fast Facts,* 351-364.

[45] Murray, ed. et al., *The PDR Pocket Guide to Prescription Drugs,* 241, 373, 443, 449, 816, 867, 908, 920, 1036, 1060, 1133, 1262, 1262, 1374, 1421.

[46] American Medical Association, ed. et al., *Essential Guide To Depression.*161-162.

[47] Maxmen, et al., *Psychotropic Drugs Fast Facts,* 351-364.

[48] M. Hiti. *New Warning on Effexor Overdoses. (FDA News Release. Oct. 17, 2006).*

[49] Murray, ed. et al., *The PDR Pocket Guide to Prescription Drugs*, 241, 373, 443, 449, 816, 867, 908, 920, 1036, 1060, 1133, 1262, 1262, 1374, 1421.

[50] American Medical Association, ed. et al., *Essential Guide To Depression.*162-165.

[51] N. L. Keltner, D.G. Folks. *Psychotropic Drugs - Third Edition.* (St. Louis, MI. Mosby, Inc. 2001) 124-165.

[52] American Medical Association, ed. et al., *Essential Guide To Depression.* 162-165156-158.

[53] Maxmen, et al., *Psychotropic Drugs Fast Facts,* 351-364.

[54] H. Miradda. *FDA Oks Abilify for Depression. (FDA News Release Nov. 20, 2007).*

[55] K. Riley. *FDA Oks TMS Depression Device. (FDA News Release. Brief Summary from the Neurological Devices Panel Meeting. Jan. 26, 2007).*

[56] Ibid.

[57] E. Turner. *Picture of Antidepressants Too Rosy? (The New England Journal of Medicine, v 358. Jan. 17, 2008)* 252-260.

[58] Murray, ed. et al., *The PDR Pocket Guide to Prescription Drugs*, 241, 373, 443, 449, 816, 867, 908, 920, 1036, 1060, 1133, 1262, 1262, 1374, 1421.

[59] M. C. Miller, ed. *Testing Antidepressants: How Methods Affect Results. (Harvard Mental Health Letter* 21:8, 2005) 7.

[60] C. Hobbs. *St. John's Wort The Mood Enhancing Herb.* (Loveland, CO: Interweave Press. 1997)16-20.

[61] Pedersen. et al. *Ginkgo: Increase Intellect and Improve Circulation.* 4-7.

[62] S. Bratman. *St. John's Wort and Depression,* (USA. Prima Publishing. 1999)4-8.

[63] Ibid, 4-8.

[64] K. Linde, et al., *St. John's Wort for Depression: An Overview and Meta-Analysis of Randomized Clinical Trials.* (*British Medical Journal* 313, 1996) 253-258.

[65] V. E. Tyler. *St. John's Wort Update: What You Need to Know About Interactions.* (*Prevention*, 52:8, 2000) 117-120.

[66] M. Angell, and J. P. Kassirer. *Alternative Medicine the Risks of Untested and Unregulated Remedies.* (*New England Journal of Medicine.* v.330, 1998) 839-841.

[67] K. Linde. *St. John's Wort for Major Depression. (The Cochrane Library. Issue 4. Oct. 7, 2008).* 1-143.

[68] Bratman, et al., *St. John's Wort and Depression*, 4-8.

[69] Gaster, et al., *St. John's Wort for Depression: A Systematic Review.* 1125.

[70] S. Foster. *101 Medicinal Herbs.* (Loveland, CO: Interweave Press. 1998)192-193.

[71] J. Brockmoller, T. Reum, S. Bauer, R. Kerb, W. D. Hubner, and I. Roots. *Hypericin and Pseudohypericin: Pharmacokinetics and the Effects on Photosensitivity in Humans.* (*Pharmacopsychiatry.* 30:2, 1997) 94-101.

[72] J. A. Henry, C.A. Alexander, and E. K. Sener. *Relative Mortality From Overdose of Antidepressants.* (*British Medical Journal,* 310, 1995)221-224.

[73] J. E. Henney. *Risk of Drug Interactions with St. John's Wort.* (*Journal of the American Medical Association.* 283:13, 2000) 1125.

[74] S. W. Lininger. *A-Z Guide to Drug-Herb-Vitamin Interactions.* (Roseville, CA: Prima Publishing. 1999)95,98,150,166,170,188,213,217.

[75] Bratman, et al., *St. John's Wort and Depression*, 4-8.

[76] Hobbs. et al., *St. John's Wort The Mood Enhancing Herb.*16-20.

[77] K. Keville. *Herbs for Health and Healing*, (Emmaus, PA: Rodale Press, Inc. 1996)30-34.

[78] P. D. Kramer. *Listening to Prozac.* (New York, NY: Penguin Books. 1994)108-116.

[79] S. Grazi, and M. Costa. *SAMe: The European Arthritis and Depression Breakthrough.* (Rocklin, CA: Prima Publishing Co. 1999)134-138.

[80] IBID, 134-138.

[81] W. Conkling. *Secrets of Ginkgo.* (New York, NY:St. Martin's Press, 1999) 9-21.

[82] Pedersen. et al., *Ginkgo: Increase Intellect and Improve Circulation.* 8-10.

[83] Conkling, et al., *Secrets of Ginkgo.* 9-21.

[84] Keville, et al., *Herbs for Health and Healing*, 30-34.

[85] Ibid, 30-34.

[86] Ibid, 30-34 .

[87] American Medical Association, ed. et al., *Essential Guide To Depression.*187-189.

[88] M. Siegel, N. Burke. *Herbs for Health and Happiness*, (Alexandria, VA: Time Life Books, 1999)94-97.

[89] Ibid,94-97.

[90] M. Evans. *The Complete Guide to Natural Remedies.*(New York, NY: Lorenz Books, 1999)121-131.

[91] L. Tenney. *Nutritional Guide A Comprehensive Reference for Better Health,* (Pleasant Grove, UT: Woodland Publishing. 1997)165-167.

[92] M. A. Brown. *When Your Body Gets The Blues.* (Emmaus, PA: Rodale Press, Inc. 2002) 91-101.

[93] U. Erasmus. *Fats that Heal, Fats That Kill.* (Burnaby BC, Canada: Alive Books, 1993)35,177,272,286,313,336.

[94] Ibid, 35,177,272,286,313,336.

[95] M. Murray, and J. Pizzorno. *Encyclopedia of Natural Medicine.* (Rocklin, CA: Prima Publishing. 1991)260-268.

[96] P. Pitchford. *Healing With Whole Foods: Oriental Traditions and Modern Nutrition.* (Berkeley, CA: North Atlantic Books. 1993)298-299.

[97] Pfeiffer, et al., *Nutrition and Mental Illness,* 26-28.

[98] Murray, et al.. *Encyclopedia of Natural Medicine.* 260-268.

[99] S. Althoff, P. N. Williams, D. Molvig, and L. Schuster. *A Guide to Alternative Medicine,* (Lincolnwood, IL: Publications International Ltd., 1997) 67-69, 203, 255-256, 280.

[100] M. Hutchison. *MegaBrain: New Tools and Techniques for Brain Growth and Mind Expansion*, (New York, NY: Ballantine Books, 1991)310-311.

[101] J. Kabot-Zinn. *Full Catastrophe Living,* (New York, NY: Dell Publishing, 1990)1-14.

[102] M. C. Miller, ed. *Meditation in Psychotherapy. (Harvard Mental Health Letter. 21-10.* April, 2005)1-3.

[103.] R. G. Meyer. *Practical Clinical Hypnosis,* (New York, NY: Lexington Books. 1992) 1-7.

CHAPTER VI:
HEADACHES & MIGRAINES

[1] S. Diamond. *Conquering Your Migraine.* (New York, NY: Simon & Schuster, 2001)19-21.

[2] A. Mauskop, and B. Fox. *What Your Doctor May Not Tell You About Migraines.* (New York, NY: Warner Books, 2001)15-25.

[3] A.M. Rapoport, and F.D. Sheftell. *Headache Relief.* (New York, NY: Fireside Books. 1991).45-55

[4] B. Tozer. *Migraine Prevention Rare in Women. (Mayo Clinic Proceedings. Vol. 81. August, 2006)* 1086-1092.

[5] M. Bigal. *Poorer Teens May Get More Migraines. (Neurology. Vol. 69. July 3, 2007)*16-25.

[6] R. Voelker. *Migraine on the Rise. (JAMA, Journal of the American Medical Association.* 282:20, 1999) 217.

[7] S. Althoff, P. N. Williams, D. Molvig, and L. Schuster, *A Guide to Alternative Medicine.* (Lincolnwood, IL: Publications International Ltd., 1997). 67-69,203,255-256,280.

8   S. Diamond. *Diagnosis of Migraines.* (*Archives of Neurology.* 8:3,1999)234-236.

9   Diamond.et al., *Conquering Your Migraine.* 22-28.

10 D. R. Goldman, and D.A. Horowitz, *American College of Physicians Home Medical Guide to Migraine & Other Headaches.* (New York, NY: Dorling Kindersley LTD. 2000)29-36.

11 Rapoport, et al., *Headache Relief.* 45-55.

12 B. S. Schwartz, W. F. Stewart, D. Simon, and R. B. Lipton. *Epidemiology of Tension-Type Headache.* (*Journal of the American Medical Association.* 279:5,1998)381-383.

13 Diamond.et al., *Conquering Your Migraine.* 22-28.

14 Diamond.et al., *Conquering Your Migraine.* 27-29.

15 Ibid, 27-29.

16 Rapoport, et al., *Headache Relief.* 47-49.

17 Diamond.et al., *Conquering Your Migraine.* 22-28.

18 N. K. Loh, D.S. Dinner, N. Foldvary, F. Skolbieranda, and W.W. Yew. *Do Patients With Obstructive Sleep Apnea Wake Up With Headaches?* (*Archives of Internal Medicine,* 159:15, 1999)1765-1768.

19 J. R. Saper. *Posttraumatic Headache A Neurobehavioral Disorder.* (*Archives of Neurology.* 57:12, 2000)118-124.

20 Rapoport, et al., *Headache Relief.* 48-81.

21 Ibid, 48-56.

22 Mauskop, et al., *What Your Doctor May Not Tell You About Migraines.* 26-27.

23 Diamond.et al., *Conquering Your Migraine.* 22-28.

24 Rapoport, et al., *Headache Relief.* 48-81.

25 Ibid, 56-80.

26 N. Hadjikhani. *Migraine Linked to Brain Lesions.* (*Neurology. Nov. 20, 2007 online source).*

27 K. Brenan. *Woman's Brain Wired for More Migraines.* (*Annals of Nuerology. Vol. 61. June 2007)* 603-606.

28 Mauskop, et al., *What Your Doctor May Not Tell You About Migraines.* 41-42.

29 Rapoport, et al., *Headache Relief.* 58-60.

30 Ibid, 58-60.

31 M. D. Eades. *The Doctor's Complete Guide To Vitamins and Minerals.* (New York, NY: Dell Publishing. 1994)315-320.

32 M. Murray, and J. Pizzorno. *Encyclopedia of Natural Medicine.* (Rocklin, CA: Prima Publishing. 1991)410-421.

33 Rapoport, et al., *Headache Relief.* 190-201.

34 L. Tenney. *Nutritional Guide A Comprehensive Reference for Better Health,* (Pleasant Grove, UT: Woodland Publishing. 1997)197-200.

[35] Rapoport, et a.., *Headache Relief.* 204-205.

[36] Mauskop, et al., *What Your Doctor May Not Tell You About Migraines.* 122-134.

[37] H. S. Smith, et al. *Do Your Sleep Habits Trigger Migraines. (Neurology. Vol. 46. 2006)*1039.

[38] Diamond.et al., *Conquering Your Migraine.* 142-154

[39] Ibid, 142-154.

[40] Althoff, et al., *A Guide to Alternative Medicine.* 67-69,203,255-256,280.

[41] Diamond.et al., *Conquering Your Migraine.* 90-93.

[42] H. Miranda. *Migraine. Depression Drugs Risky Mix. (FDA News Release, July 19, 2006)*

[43] Mauskop, et al., *What Your Doctor May Not Tell You About Migraines.* 171-208.

[44] L. Murray, ed. *The PDR Pocket Guide to Prescription Drugs*, (New York, NY: Simon & Schuster. Inc. 2008) 116, 119, 187, 291, 1382.

[45] H. M. Lyman, C. Fenger, H. W. Jones, and W. T. Belfield. *The New American Family Physician.* (Chicago,Il: Reilly & Britton Co. 1905)340.

[46] Diamond.et a.., *Conquering Your Migraine.* 90-93.

[47] Mauskop, et al., *What Your Doctor May Not Tell You About Migraines.* 171-208.

[48] Murray, ed. et al., *The PDR Pocket Guide to Prescription Drugs*, 116, 119, 187, 291, 1382.

[49] Althoff, et al., *A Guide to Alternative Medicine.* 67-69,203,255-256,280.

[50] Mauskop, et al., *What Your Doctor May Not Tell You About Migraines.* 36-54.

[51] Ibid, 38-53.

[52] D.G. Williams. *The Top Three Migraine Cures From Around the World*, (*Alternative For The Health-Conscious Individual.* Sp. Report, 2001)1-2.

[53] Althoff, et al., *A Guide to Alternative Medicine.* 67-69,203,255-256,280.

[54] S. Foster. *101 Medicinal Herbs.* (Loveland, CO: Interweave Press. 1998)86-87.

[55] J. Carper. *Miracle Cures.* (New York, NY: Harper Collins Publishers. 1997)83-90.

[56] Mauskop. et al., *What Your Doctor May Not Tell You About Migraines.* 36-54.

[57] Ibid, 40-54.

[58] Ibid, 44-54.

[59] Murray, et al., *Encyclopedia of Natural Medicine.* 260-268.

[60] C. C. Pfeiffer. *Nutrition and Mental Illness*, (Rochester, VT: Healing Arts Press. 1987)101.

[61] Rapoport, et al., *Headache Relief.* 212-214.

[62] Tenney, et al., *Nutritional Guide A Comprehensive Reference for Better Health,* 197-200.

[63] Eades, et al., *The Doctor's Complete Guide To Vitamins and Minerals.* 315-320.

[64] E. M. Haas. *Staying Healthy with Nutrition.* (Berkeley, CA: Celestial Arts. 1992)67-68.

[65] P. Pitchford. *Healing With Whole Foods: Oriental Traditions and Modern Nutrition.* (Berkeley, CA: North Atlantic Books. 1993)126-135.

[66] Althoff, et al., *A Guide to Alternative Medicine.* 67-69,203,255-256,280.

[67] Foster, et al., *101 Medicinal Herbs.* 76-77.

[68] S. W. Lininger. *A-Z Guide to Drug-Herb-Vitamin Interactions.* (Roseville, CA: Prima Publishing. 1999)34,62,84,85,170,173.

[69] P. A. Balch. *Prescription For Herbal Healing,* (New York, NY: Avery Books. 2002)353-355.

[70] Foster, et al., *101 Medicinal Herbs.* 188-189.

[71] Balch, et al., *Prescription For Herbal Healing,* 353-355.

[72] Foster, et al., *101 Medicinal Herbs.* 210-211.

[73] M. Siegel, and N. Burke. *Herbs for Health and Happiness,* (Alexandria, VA: Time Life Books. 1999)14-17.

[74] Balch, et al., *Prescription For Herbal Healing,* 353-355.

[75] Lininger, et al., *A-Z Guide to Drug-Herb-Vitamin Interactions.* 34, 62, 84, 85, 170, 173.

[76] Balch, et al., *Prescription For Herbal Healing,* 353-355.

[77] Williams, et al., *The Top Three Migraine Cures From Around the World,* 1-2.

[78] M. Evans. *The Complete Guide to Natural Remedies,* (New York, NY: Lorenz Books, 1999)121-131.

[79] M. Lavabre. *Aromatherapy Workbook,* (Rochester, VT: Healing Arts Press, 1990)75,83-85,102.

[80] Althoff, et al., *A Guide to Alternative Medicine.* 67-69,203,255-256,280.

[81] Diamond.et al. *Conquering Your Migraine.* 187.

[82] B. Burns. *New Treatment for Cluster Headaches. (The Lancet, March 8, 2007. Online edition).*

[83] Y. Mohammad. *Pulse Away Migraine Pain.* American Headache Society annual scientific meeting, Boston, MA, June 26-29, 2008.

[84] M. Hutchison, *MegaBrain: New Tools and Techniques for Brain Growth and Mind Expansion,* (New York, NY: Ballantine Books, 1991)310-311.

[85] Murray, et al. *Encyclopedia of Natural Medicine.* 260-268.

[86] Althoff, et al. *A Guide to Alternative Medicine.* 67-69,203,255-256,280.

[87] Diamond, et al., *Conquering Your Migraine.* 185-186.

[88] Murray, et al., *Encyclopedia of Natural Medicine.* 260-268.

89 C. Dahlof. *Migraines May Ease with Age. (Headache. Vol. 46, October, 2006)* s144-s146.

CHAPTER VII:
OTHER DISORDERS

1 N. L. Keltner, D.G. Folks. *Psychotropic Drugs - Third Edition.* (St. Louis,MI. Mosby, Inc. 2001) 122-128.

2 Ibid, 1254-125.

3 E.M. Frams. *Bipolar Risk for Kids Born to Older Dads. (Archives of General Psychiatry. Vol. 65. September, 2008)* 1034-1040.

4 P. Lichtenstein. *Schizophrenia, Bipolar Disorder. Gene Link? (The Lancet. Vol. 373. January 17, 2009)*234-239.

5 American Psychiatric Association, *The Diagnostic and Statistical Manual of Mental Disorders, 4th edition, Text Revision,* (Washington, DC: American Psychiatric Association, 2000) 345-368.

6 Ibid, 345-368.

7 Ibid, 345-368.

8 Ibid, 345-368.

9 Ibid, 369-376.

10 N. L. Keltner, D.G. Folks. *Psychotropic Drugs - Third Edition.* (St. Louis,MI. Mosby, Inc. 2001)128.

11 L. Murray, ed. *The PDR Pocket Guide to Prescription Drugs,* (New York, NY: Simon & Schuster, Inc. 2008)544-547.

12 Ibid, 1636-1637.

13 Ibid, 425-425.

14 Ibid, 1367-1371.

15 W. Conkling. *Secrets of Ginseng.* (New York, NY: St. Martin's Paperbacks. 1999)58-60.

16 M. Siegel, and N. Burke. *Herbs for Health and Happiness,* (Alexandria, VA: Time Life Books. 1995)95-96.

17 Siegel, et al., *Herbs for Health and Happiness,* 95-96.

18 Ibid, 95-96.

19 Ibid, 93-96.

20 Ibid, 93-96.

21 R. Somerville. ed. *The Drug and Natural Medicine Advisor.* (Richmond, VI: Time-Life Books. 1997)195-196.

22 Somerville. ed. et al., *The Drug and Natural Medicine Advisor.* 461.

23 N. L. Keltner, D.G. Folks. *Psychotropic Drugs - Third Edition.* 78-86.

[24] American Psychiatric Association, *The Diagnostic and Statistical Manual of Mental Disorders, 4th edition, Text Revision.* 297-311.

[25] N. L. Keltner, D.G. Folks. *Psychotropic Drugs - Third Edition.* 83-86.

[26] C. Pfeiffer. *Nutrition and Mental Illness.* (Rochester, VT: Healing arts Press. 1987) 3-17.

[27] S. Saha. *Schizophrenia Rarer Than Previously Thought. (Public Library of Science Medicine. Vol. 2. May, 2005)*413-433.

[28] H. W. Griffith. *Complete Guide to Prescription & Nonprescription Drugs.* (New York, NY: The Berkley Publishing Group. 2004).

[29] C. Pfeiffer. *Nutrition and Mental Illness.* 9-11.

[30] T. Lencz. *New DNA Clue for Schizophrenia. (Molecular Psychiatry, March, 2007)* online edition.

[31] S. Bahn. *Schizophrenia, Bipolar May Share Cause. (The Lancet, vol. 362. Sept. 5, 2003)* 787-805.

[32] A. Brown. *Schizophrenia Linked to Flu During Pregnancy. (Archives of General Psychiatry, vol. 61. August, 2004)* 774-780.

[33] S. G. Birnbaum. *Bipolar Disorder, Schizophrenia Key Found. (Science, vol. 306, Oct. 2004)* 882-884.

[34] E. Messias. *Summer Birth Linked To Type of Schizophrenia. (Archives of General Psychiatry, vol. 81, Oct. 2004)* 983-989.

[35] W. Eaton. *Gluten Intolerance Linked to Schizophrenia. (British Medical Journal, vol. 328, Feb. 21, 2004)* 438-439.

[36] C. Pfeiffer. *Nutrition and Mental Illness.* 18-25.

[37] Ibid. 26-32.

[38] Ibid. 33-47.

[39] Ibid. 48-52.

[40] Ibid. 57-65.

[41] Ibid. 33-47.

[42] Ibid. 48-52.

[43] Ibid. 57-65.

[44] M. Siegel, and N. Burke. *Herbs for Health and Happiness,* (Alexandria, VA: Time Life Books. 1999)95-96.

CHAPTER VIII:
SPIRITUAL HEALING

See Suggested Further Reading

CHAPTER IX:
Conclusions

1   American Psychiatric Association. *Diagnostic and Statistical Manual of Mental Disorders-Fourth Edition-Text Revision,* Washington, DC: APA. 2000) 154-156.

2   J .S. Bland. *Genetic Nutritioneering,* (Los Angeles, CA: Keats Publishing. 1999) 104-106.

3   J. Lombard, and C. Germano. *The Brain Wellness Plan,* (New York, NY: Kensington Books. 1997)65.

4   C. W. Henderson. *On-The-Job Lead Exposure Could Increase Risk.* (Medical Letter on the CDC & FDA. 2000)1.

5   Mayo Clinic ed. *Successful Aging,* (Rochester, MN: Mayo Foundation. 2000)3-4.

6   R. Mayeux, and M. Sano. *Treatment of Alzheimer's Disease,* (*The New England Journal of Medicine.* v22, 1999)167.

7   L. Murray, ed. *The PDR Pocket Guide to Prescription Drugs,* (New York, NY: Simon & Schuster, Inc. 2008) 96, 275, 491.

8   J. R. T. Davidson, and K. M. Connor.. *Herbs for the Mind,* (New York, NY: The Guilford Press. 2000) 159-162.

9   Ibid, 161-162.

10 S. W. Lininger. *A-Z Guide to Drug-Herb-Vitamin Interactions,* (Roseville, CA: Prima Publishing. 1999)95,98.

11 Ibid, 225-226.

12 L. G. Miller. *Selected Clinical Consideration Focusing on Known or Potential Drug-Herb Interactions,* (JAMA: *Journal of The American Medical Association.* v158:20, 1998) 125-1127.

13 V. E. Tyler. *Herbal Hope for Alzheimer's, Cancer, and Prostrate Disease,* (*Prevention.* v53:3, 2001)105-106.

14 R. Lethem, and M. Orrell. *Antioxidants and Dementia,* (*The Lancet.* v349, 1997) 1189.

15 E. Mindell. *Earl Mindell's Food as Medicine,* (New York, NY: Simon & Schuster. 1994)68.

16 L. Tenney. *Nutritional Guide A Comprehensive Reference for Better Health,* (Pleasant Grove, UT: Woodland Publishing. 1997)115.

17 Lombard, et al., *The Brain Wellness Plan.* 70-71.

18 Ibid, 72-73.

19 D. S .Pine, ed. *Fluvoxamine for the Treatment of Anxiety Disorder in Children and Adolescents.* (*New England Journal of Medicine.*v.344:17 2001)1279-1285.

[20] American Psychiatric Association. ed. et al., *Diagnostic and Statistical Manual of Mental Disorders-Fourth Edition-Text Revision,* 429-430.

[21] D. R. Weinberger. *Anxiety at the Frontier of Molecular Medicine. (New England Journal of Medicine.* v.3442001)1247-1249.

[22] P. D. Kramer. *Listening to Prozac.* (New York, NY: Penguin Books.1994)101.

[23] Ibid, 103.

[24] C. C. Pfeiffer. *Nutrition and Mental Illness,* (Rochester, VT: Healing Arts Press. 1987)26-28.

[25] P. A. Balch. *Prescription For Herbal Healing,* (New York, NY: Avery Books. 2002)190-191.

[26] Murray, ed. et al., *The PDR Pocket Guide to Prescription Drugs,* 116, 119, 187, 291, 1382.

[27] J. S. Maxmen, and N.G. Ward. *Psychotropic Drugs Fast Facts,* (New York, NY: W.W. Norton & Company. 1995)255-309.

[28] W. Conkling. *Secrets of Ginseng.* (New York, NY: St. Martin's Paperbacks. 1999)58-60.

[29] M. Siegel, and N. Burke. *Herbs for Health and Happiness,* (Alexandria, VA: Time Life Books. 1999)95-96.

[30] Ibid, 93-99.

[31] M. D. Eades. *The Doctor's Complete Guide To Vitamins and Minerals.* (New York, NY: Dell Publishing. 1994)464-466.

[32] E. M. Haas. *Staying Healthy with Nutrition.* (Berkeley, CA: Celestial Arts. 1992)740-741.

[33] Mindell, et al., *Earl Mindell's Food as Medicine,* 238-240.

[34] M. Murray, and J. Pizzorno. *Encyclopedia of Natural Medicine.* (Rocklin, CA: Prima Publishing. 1991)91-99.

[35] P. Pitchford. *Healing With Whole Foods: Oriental Traditions and Modern Nutrition.* (Berkeley, CA: North Atlantic Books. 1993)179.

[36] Tenney,. et al., *Nutritional Guide A Comprehensive Reference for Better Health,* 273-275.

[37] Balch, et al., *Prescription For Herbal Healing,* 190-191.

[38] S. Althoff, P. N. Williams, D. Molvig, and L. Schuster. *A Guide to Alternative Medicine,* (Lincolnwood, IL: Publications International Ltd., 1997)31-34.

[39] M. Hutchison. *MegaBrain: New Tools and Techniques for Brain Growth and Mind Expansion,* (New York, NY: Ballantine Books, 1991)270-273.

[40] M. Evans. *The Complete Guide to Natural Remedies,* (New York, NY: Lorenz Books, 1999)91-101.

[41] M. Lavabre. *Aromatherapy Workbook,* (Rochester, VT: Healing Arts Press, 1990)77,82,85,88.

[42] American Academy of Pediatrics (2000, May1). AAP Releases New Guidelines For Diagnosis of ADHD. (Press release posted on the World Wide Web) AAP author. Retrieved June 1, 2000 WWW:http://www.aap. org/advocacy/releases/mayadhd.htm.

[43] K. S. Berger. *The Developing Person Through the Life Span.* (New York, NY: Worth Publishers,1998)318-321.

[44] Lombard, et al., *The Brain Wellness Plan.* 151-161

[45] B. F. Feingold *Why Your Child Is Hyperactive.* (New York, NY: Random House, 1975)15-18.

[46] M. Bricklin. *The Practical Encyclopedia of Natural Healing.* (Emmaus, PE:
Rodale Press, 1983)101.

[47] D. S. Nambudripad. *Say Good-bye To ADD and ADHD.* (Buena park, CA: Delta Publishing Co. 1999)76-77.

[48] S. Weintraub. *Natural Treatments for ADD and Hyperactivity,* (Pleasant Grove, UT: Woodland Publishing, 1997)121-128.

[49] M. A. Block. *No More Ritalin: Treating ADHD Without Drugs,* (New York, NY: Kensington Publishing Corp. 1996)74-79.

[50] Lombard, et al., *The Brain Wellness Plan.* 158-161.

[51] Murray, ed. et al., *The PDR Pocket Guide to Prescription Drugs,* 27, 325, 378, 1092.

[52] Maxmen, et al , *Psychotropic Drugs Fast Facts,* 351-364.

[53] Feingold, et al., *Why Your Child Is Hyperactive.* 16-18.

[54] Bricklin, et al., *The Practical Encyclopedia of Natural Healing.* 101.

[55] Mindell, et al., *Earl Mindell's Food as Medicine,* 238-240.

[56] Eades, et al., *The Doctor's Complete Guide To Vitamins and Minerals.* 464-466.

[57] Block, et al., *No More Ritalin: Treating ADHD Without Drugs,* 74-79.

[58] Nambudripad, et al., *Say Good-bye To ADD and ADHD.* 76-77.

[59] Weintraub, et al., *Natural Treatments for ADD and Hyperactivity,* 121-128.

[60] M. Salaman. *Foods That Heal.* (Menlo Park, CA: Statford Pub. 1989)98-101.

[61] Weintraub, et al., *Natural Treatments for ADD and Hyperactivity,* 121-128.

[62] R. J. Goldberg. *Depression in the Workplace: Economics and Interventions,* (Behavioral Healthcare Tomorrow 10:6, 2001, 10-11.

[63] American Psychiatric Association. ed. *Diagnostic and Statistical Manual of Mental Disorders-Fourth Edition-Text Revision,* (Washington, DC: APA. 2000)369-380.

[64] B. Birmaher, N. Ryan, D.E. Willianson, D.A. Brent, J. Kaufman, R.E.

Dahl, J. Perel, B. Nelson. *Childhood and Adolescent Depression: A Review of the Past 10 Years.* (Journal of the American Academy of Child and Adolescent Psychiatry 35:11, 1996) 1427-1428.

[65] American Psychiatric Association. et al., *Diagnostic and Statistical Manual of Mental Disorders-Fourth Edition-Text Revision.* 369-380.

[66] American Medical Association, ed. *Essential Guide To Depression.* (New York: Pocket Books, 1980) 21-31.

[67] Birmaher, et al., *Childhood and Adolescent Depression: A Review of the Past 10 Years.* 1427-1428.

[68] Tenney, et al., *Nutritional Guide A Comprehensive Reference for Better Health,* 165-166.

[69] American Medical Association, ed. et al., *Essential Guide To Depression.* 21-31.

[70] Ibid, 21-31.

[71] Maxmen, et al., *Psychotropic Drugs Fast Facts,* 351-364.

[72] N. L. Keltner, D.G. Folks. *Psychotropic Drugs - Third Edition.* (St. Louis,MI. Mosby, Inc. 2001) 127-165.

[73] Maxmen, et al. *Psychotropic Drugs Fast Facts,* 351-364.

[74] Ibid, 351-364.

[75] Murray, ed. et al., *The PDR Pocket Guide to Prescription Drugs,* 241, 373, 443, 449, 816, 867, 908, 920, 1036, 1060, 1133, 1262, 1262, 1374, 1421.

[76] Maxmen, et al., *Psychotropic Drugs Fast Facts,* 351-364.

[77] American Medical Association, ed. et al., *Essential Guide To Depression.* 21-31.

[78] Ibid, 21-31.

[79] Ibid, 21-31.

[80] Maxmen, et al., *Psychotropic Drugs Fast Facts,* 351-364.

[81] Murray, ed. et al., *The PDR Pocket Guide to Prescription Drugs,* 241, 373, 443, 449, 816, 867, 908, 920, 1036, 1060, 1133, 1262, 1262, 1374, 1421.

[82] B. Gaster, and J. Holroyd. *St. John's Wort for Depression: A Systematic Review.* (*New England Journal of Medicine* 160:2, 2000)1125.

[83] S. Bratman. *St. John's Wort and Depression,* (USA. Prima Publishing. 1999)4-8.

[84] V. E. Tyler. *St. John's Wort Update: What You Need to Know About Interactions.* (*Prevention,* 52:8, 2000) 117-120.

[85] J. E. Henney. *Risk of Drug Interactions with St. John's Wort.* (*Journal of the American Medical Association.* 283:13, 2000) 1125.

[86] S. W. Lininger. *A-Z Guide to Drug-Herb-Vitamin Interactions.* (Roseville, CA: Prima Publishing. 1999)95,98,150,166,170,188,213,217.

[87] J. A. Henry, C.A. Alexander, and E. K. Sener *Relative Mortality From Overdose of Antidepressants.* (*British Medical Journal*, 310, 1995)221-224.

[88] W. Conkling. *Secrets of Ginkgo.* (New York, NY:St. Martin's Press, 1999) 9-21.

[89] S. Pedersen. *Ginkgo: Increase Intellect and Improve Circulation.* (New York, NY: Dorling Kindersley Publishing Co. 2000) 4-14,32-34.

[90] American Medical Association, ed. et al., *Essential Guide To Depression.* 21-31.

[91] W. Conkling. *Secrets of Ginseng.* (New York, NY: St. Martin's Paperbacks, 1999)52-59.

[92] K. Keville. *Herbs for Health and Healing,* (Emmaus, PA: Rodale Press, Inc. 1996)30-34.

[93] S. Pedersen. *Kava: Relax Your Muscles & Mind,* (New York, NY: Dorling Kindersley Publishing Co. 2000) 22-24.

[94] M. Siegel, and N. Burke. *Herbs for Health and Happiness,* (Alexandria, VA: Time Life Books, 1999)94-97.

[95] Williams, et al., *The Top Three Migraine Cures From Around the World,* 1-2.

[96] Keltner et al., *Psychotropic Drugs - Third Edition,* 127-165.

[97] Tenney, et al., *Nutritional Guide A Comprehensive Reference for Better Health,* 165-167.

[98] M. A. Brown. *When Your Body Gets The Blues.* (Emmaus, PA: Rodale Press, Inc. 2002) 91-101.

[99] U. Erasmus. *Fats that Heal, Fats That Kill.* (Burnaby BC, Canada: Alive Books, 1993)35,177,272,286,313,336.

[100] Murray, et al., *Encyclopedia of Natural Medicine.* 260-268.

[101] Ibid, 260-268.

[102] Althoff, et al., *A Guide to Alternative Medicine.* 67-69,203,255-256,280.

[103] Hutchison, et al., *MegaBrain: New Tools and Techniques for Brain Growth and Mind Expansion.* 310-311.

[104] S. Diamond. *Conquering Your Migraine.* (New York, NY: Simon & Schuster, 2001)19-21.

[105] D. R. Goldman, and D. A. Horowitz. *American College of Physicians Home Medical Guide to Migraine & Other Headaches.* (New York, NY: Dorling Kindersley LTD. 2000)29-36.

[106] Diamond.et al., *Conquering Your Migraine.* 22-28.

[107] A.M. Rapoport, and F.D. Sheftell. *Headache Relief.* (New York, NY: Fireside Books. 1991).45-55

[108] N. K. Loh, D.S. Dinner, N. Foldvary, F. Skolbieranda, and W.W. Yew. *Do Patients With Obstructive Sleep Apnea Wake Up With Headaches?* (*Archives of Internal Medicine,* 159:15, 1999)1765-1768.

[109] A. Mauskop, and B. Fox. *What Your Doctor May Not Tell You About Migraines.* (New York, NY: Warner Books, 2001)15-25.

[110] Rapoport, et al., *Headache Relief.* 45-55.

[111] Ibid, 45-55.

[112] Mauskop, et al., *What Your Doctor May Not Tell You About Migraines.* 15-25.

[113] Eades, et al., *The Doctor's Complete Guide To Vitamins and Minerals.* 315-320.

[114] Murray, et al., *Encyclopedia of Natural Medicine.* 410-421.

[115] Tenney, et al., *Nutritional Guide A Comprehensive Reference for Better Health,* 197-200.

[116] Diamond. et al., *Conquering Your Migraine.* 35-37.

[117] Althoff, et al., *A Guide to Alternative Medicine.* 67-69,203,255-256,280.

[118] Diamond.et al., *Conquering Your Migraine.* 142-151.

[119] Mauskop, et al., *What Your Doctor May Not Tell You About Migraines.* 171-176.

[120] Murray, ed. et al., *The PDR Pocket Guide to Prescription Drugs.* 68, 190, 366, 599, 607, 720, 762, 764, 1425.

[121] Althoff, et al., *A Guide to Alternative Medicine.* 67-69,203,255-256,280.

[122] Mauskop, et al., *What Your Doctor May Not Tell You About Migraines.* 37-53.

[123] D. G. Williams. *The Top Three Migraine Cures From Around the World,* (*Alternative For The Health-Conscious Individual.* Sp. Report, 2001)1-2.

[124] J. Carper. *Miracle Cures.* (New York, NY: Harper Collins Publishers. 1997)83-90.

[125] S. Foster. *101 Medicinal Herbs.* (Loveland, CO: Interweave Press. 1998)86-87.

[126] Murray, et al., *Encyclopedia of Natural Medicine.* 410-421.

[127] Pfeiffer, et al., *Nutrition and Mental Illness,* 101.

[128] Rapoport, et al., *Headache Relief.* 212-214.

[129] Tenney, et al., *Nutritional Guide A Comprehensive Reference for Better Health,* 197-200.

[130] Eades, et al., *The Doctor's Complete Guide To Vitamins and Minerals.* 315-320.

[131] Althoff, et al. *A Guide to Alternative Medicine.* 67-69,203,255-256,280.

[132] Murray, et al., *Encyclopedia of Natural Medicine.* 410-421.

[133] Foster, et al., *101 Medicinal Herbs.* 86-87.

[134] Balch, et al., *Prescription For Herbal Healing,* 353-355.

[135] Pitchford, et al., *Healing With Whole Foods: Oriental Traditions and Modern Nutrition.* 126-135.

[136] Siegel, et al., *Herbs for Health and Happiness,* 14-17.

[137] Evans, et al., *The Complete Guide to Natural Remedies*.121-131.

[138] Lavabre, et al., *Aromatherapy Workbook*. 75,83-86,102.

[139] Diamond.et al., *Conquering Your Migraine*. 121-134.

[140] Hutchison, et al., *MegaBrain: New Tools and Techniques for Brain Growth and Mind Expansion*. 310-311.

[141] Althoff, et al., *A Guide to Alternative Medicine*. 67-69,203,255-256,280.

[142] Murray, et al., *Encyclopedia of Natural Medicine*. 410-421.

[143] Mauskop, et al., *What Your Doctor May Not Tell You About Migraines*. 37-53.

[144] Williams, et al., *The Top Three Migraine Cures From Around the World*, 1-2.

[145] N. L. Keltner, D.G. Folks. *Psychotropic Drugs - Third Edition*. (St. Louis,MI. Mosby, Inc. 2001) 122-128.

[146] Ibid, 1254-125.

[147] H. W. Griffith. *Complete Guide to Prescription & Nonprescription Drugs*. (New York, NY: The Berkley Publishing Group. 2004).

[148] M. Siegel, and N. Burke. *Herbs for Health and Happiness*, (Alexandria, VA: Time Life Books. 1999)95-96.

[149] American Psychiatric Association, *The Diagnostic and Statistical Manual of Mental Disorders, 4th edition, Text Revision*, (Washington, DC: American Psychiatric Association, 2000).

[150] N. L. Keltner, D.G. Folks. *Psychotropic Drugs - Third Edition*. (St. Louis,MI. Mosby, Inc. 2001).

[151] C. Pfeiffer. *Nutrition and Mental Illness*. (Rochester, VT: Healing arts Press. 1987) 3-17.

[152] Murray, ed. et al., *The PDR Pocket Guide to Prescription Drugs*, 116, 119, 187, 291, 1382.

[153] Maxmen, et al., *Psychotropic Drugs Fast Facts*, 255-309.

[154] B. Goldberg. *The Science of Deceit*, (*Alternative Medicine* v.46, 2002)12-15.

[155] A. Hofffer, and M. Walker. *Orthomolecular Nutrition*. (New Canaan, CT: Keats Publishing, 1978)181-187.

[156] Pedersen, et al., *Ginkgo: Increase Intellect and Improve Circulation*. 8.

[157] Davidson, et al., *Herbs for the Mind*. 1-11.

INDEX

Migra-Lieve, 130
Miller, M.C., 207, 217, 219, 225
Mindell, E., 71, 208, 211, 214, 225, 226, 227
Mirtazapine, 88
Moban, 162, 163, 190
Moclobemide, 92
Molindone, 162, 163, 190
Molvig, D., 204, 211, 219, 226
Moran, M., 206
Motz, Julie, 174
Murray, M., 103, 206, 209, 210, 211, 213, 214, 216, 217, 219, 220, 221, 222, 223, 225, 226, 227, 228, 229, 230, 231
Myproic acid, 151
Myss, Caroline, 173, 201

N

Nadolol, 125
Nambudripad, D.S., 71, 200, 204, 213, 214, 227
Naprosen, 17
Naproxen, 15, 17, 27, 126
Nardil, 19, 41, 92, 125, 127
National Association of School Psychologists (NASP), 59
National Institutes of Health, 94
Navane, 162, 163, 190
Nefazodone, 39, 88, 93
Neroli, 48, 101
Neurofribrillary tangles, 11
Neurology, 20, 113, 206, 207, 219, 220, 221
Neuropeptides, 79
New age, xii, 174
Newton, Michael, 177, 178, 196
Niacin (B3), 22, 141
nicotine, 103, 143, 192, 193
Nifedipine, 97

Nonhydrazine, 92
Norepinephine, 78
Norpramin, 67, 73, 183
Nortriptyline, 87
Novo-doxepin, 91
Novotriptyn, 91

O

Obsessive-compulsive disorder (OCD), 31
O'Donnell, S.A., 210
Olanzapine, 151, 162, 189, 190
Omega-3, 23, 28, 34, 45, 51, 53, 61, 74, 102, 131, 141, 192
opioids, 34, 140, 188
OTC, 4, 6, 17, 122, 140, 143, 188

P

Pamelor, 91, 124
pancreas, 83, 101, 119, 125, 127, 139, 187
Panic disorder, 34, 36, 51
Pantothenic acid, 53, 141, 182
Parnate, 92
Paroxetine, 39, 92, 124
Passionflower, Passiflora incarnata, 44, 153
Pauling, Linus, 5
Paxil, 1, 36, 39, 65, 88, 92, 124
Pearl, Eric, 174, 201
Pedersen, S., 200, 204, 207, 217, 218, 229, 231
pelargonium, 101
Pemoline, 67, 214
Peppermint, 134, 142, 143, 188, 194
Perphenazine, 162, 163, 190
Pfeiffer, Carl, 12, 33, 63, 71, 85, 161, 164, 165, 166, 168, 190, 201, 205, 207, 209,

www.ingramcontent.com/pod-product-compliance
Lightning Source LLC
Chambersburg PA
CBHW061343280526
45784CB00001B/112